# A Woman's Guide

## to

# Coping with Disability

*Resources for Rehabilitation*
*Lexington, Massachusetts*

Resources for Rehabilitation
33 Bedford Street, Suite 19A
Lexington, MA 02173
(617) 862-6455

A Woman's Guide to Coping with Disability -- 2nd edition

ISBN  0-929718-19-4

Resources for Rehabilitation is a nonprofit organization dedicated to providing training and information to professionals and the public about the needs of individuals with disabilities and the resources available to meet those needs.

Library of Congress Cataloging-in-Publication Data

A woman's guide to coping with disability -- 2nd ed.
  p.  cm.
Includes bibliographical references and index.
ISBN 0-929718-19-4 (pbk.)
1. Physically handicapped women--Health and hygiene
2. Physically handicapped women--Social conditions
3. Adjustment (Psychology)   I. Resources for Rehabilitation (Organization)
RA778.W718   1997
362.4'082--dc21                                    96-51596
                                                      CIP

# TABLE OF CONTENTS

# INTRODUCTION

Information can be empowering. For women with disabilities, information can mean the difference between independence and dependence. Having accurate knowledge about programs that provide rehabilitation, training, and special equipment may enable women who would otherwise be institutionalized to live in the community, raise a family, and continue in a career. Knowledge of legal rights and opportunities is essential in our bureaucratic society.

*A Woman's Guide to Coping with Disability* provides essential information so that women may pursue their rights and obtain the services that enable them to be independent. In addition to providing information that is applicable to any woman with a disability or chronic condition, the book covers conditions that are most prevalent in women and those that are likely to affect women's special roles in society and unique physical functions, such as childbearing. Family members and service providers will also find the book to be extremely useful in their search for appropriate services. Because women have different lifestyles, needs, and degrees of impairment, the book is organized so that each woman may select the resources that are most appropriate to her own specific needs.

Each chapter includes an introductory narrative, information about national organizations that provide services to women with disabilities and chronic conditions, and information about relevant publications and tapes. Chapters 1, 2, and 3, "Women and Disability," "Coping with Daily Activities," and "Laws that Affect Women with Disabilities" provide information that is useful no matter what disability or condition interests the reader.

Beginning with Chapter 4, each chapter has introductory material describing causes and effects of a specific condition; effects of the condition on sexual functioning, pregnancy, and childrearing; psychological aspects; information on professional service providers and where to find services; major organizations serving women with the condition; and publications and tapes. Descriptions of organizations, publications and tapes, and assistive devices are alphabetical within sections. Although many of the publications described are available in libraries or bookstores, the addresses and phone numbers of publishers and distributors are included for those who wish to purchase the books by mail or phone. Only directories that have timely information and those that are updated regularly are included. Some books that are out of print are included; these may be located in libraries or bookstores that specialize in locating out of print books. Unless otherwise noted, all videotapes are produced in VHS format. Developments in computer technology, such as bulletin boards, e-mail, and the Internet, have greatly increased access to information for the general population as well as people with disabilities. E-mail and Internet addresses are given for many organizations listed in this book. Since changes and additions are frequent, readers should check bulletin boards regularly for updates.

All of the material is up-to-date, and prices were accurate at the time of publication. All prices are in U.S. dollars unless otherwise noted. However, it is always advisable to contact publishers and manufacturers to inquire about availability and current prices.

The phone numbers of organizations that have special telephone access for people with hearing or speech impairments, formerly called telecommunications devices for the deaf (TDD), are now called text telephones (TT). When organizations have these special devices, the phone number is followed by the notation "(TT)." When the same number is available for either voice or text telephone access, "(V/TT)" appears after the phone number. FAX numbers are also included when available. Phone numbers that begin with either (800) or (888) are toll-free.

# KEY TO ABBREVIATIONS AND TERMINOLOGY

BBS = bulletin board service accessible with a computer, modem, telephone line, and communication software

PC = personal computer (IBM or compatible)

TT = text telephone, special telephone system for individuals who are deaf or have hearing impairments and those who have speech impairments (formerly known as TDD, telecommunication device for the deaf)

V/TT = same telephone number for voice or text telephone

The following are terms used in relation to computer and Internet resources:

e-mail (electronic mail address)
gopher
http://
telnet
www (World Wide Web)

# Chapter 1

# WOMEN AND DISABILITY

Over the years, little attention has been paid to the special needs of women with disabilities. Just as those who conduct research in the area of health have historically omitted women from major studies, both researchers and practitioners in the areas of disability and rehabilitation have failed to address the special needs of women with disabilities. A survey of the literature prior to 1985 reveals a dearth of information about women and disability. In the middle of the 1980's, several anthologies were produced addressing this topic and lamenting the lack of attention paid to women's needs (see, for example, Deegan and Brooks: 1985; Fine and Asch: 1988). Virtually all of these collections discussed women as having double disabilities or handicaps, since women's lower status in society was also viewed as a handicap.

Numerous writers have asserted that disabilities are more difficult for women than for men. Fine and Asch (1985) present this point of view, claiming that women are less likely to receive rehabilitation training for paid positions than men; have lower self-esteem than men with disabilities; are "roleless;" and have no role models to emulate. However, Bonwich's (1985) study of women with spinal cord injuries concludes that disability actually resulted in "role expansion;" that is, women were successful in carrying out extremely difficult roles and also had opportunities for education through the vocational rehabilitation system that they would not have had otherwise.

Despite the different interpretations made by these writers, it is apparent that women with disabilities have special needs. From both a statistical perspective and a substantive perspective, the needs of women with disabilities merit much greater attention than they have received. Women constitute 53.1% of the 48.9 million Americans with disabilities; 20.2% of women have disabilities compared to 18.7% of men. Women 65 years or older have the highest rate of disability: 56.0% have disabilities, and 37.4% have severe disabilities. Just over half (50.9%) of men in this age range have disabilities. Thus, while women live longer than men, they are more likely to be disabled (McNeil: 1993).

Women play different roles in society than men and thus experience different consequences of disabilities. They are usually the nurturers in our society, providing most of the care for children, elders, and those who are sick. In addition to affecting their caregiving roles, disabilities and chronic conditions often affect the health of women during pregnancy and the health of the fetus. In recent years, most women have expanded their roles to include work outside the home, thus increasing their responsibilities. Balancing family and work can be challenging for any woman, but those with disabilities must seek out innovative solutions to the additional problems caused by their conditions.

## WOMEN AND THE HEALTH CARE SYSTEM

The American health care system has always been dominated by men. Until recently, it was rare for a woman to be admitted to medical school, and the few who were admitted experienced the same type of sexism as women patients. Recent articles, some written by women medical students and physicians themselves, reveal how medical textbooks regularly omit the effects of common conditions on women, the disparagement of female medical students by faculty members, and the sexist and debasing language used by male physicians. Until recently, women were systematically excluded from most research studies sponsored by the National Institutes of Health (NIH). To remedy this situation, the NIH Revitalization Act of 1993 (P.L. 103-42) mandates inclusion of women and minorities in research projects sponsored by NIH.

It is common for physicians to assume that women's health complaints are psychosomatic, whereas men's health complaints are assumed to have a physiological basis. Such an assumption not only results in the prescription of unnecessary mood altering drugs for women (Correa: 1975; Howell: 1976), but also may result in missing the diagnoses of serious illness. Numerous studies have documented the differential treatment the health care system provides based on gender. One study of male physicians who treated men and women for five common complaints (back pain, headache, dizziness, chest pain, and fatigue) found that men received more extensive workups than women, suggesting that the physicians took the men's complaints more seriously and viewed the women as hypochondriacal (Armitage et al.: 1979).

Despite the documented findings of sexism practiced by many physicians, women make 50% more visits to physicians than men (DeLozier and Gagnon: 1991). Older women are the most frequent consumers of health services, yet physicians are often uninterested in their needs and overprescribe medications instead of seeking the physiological source of their problems. Raised in a generation that taught them to accept authority without question, older women are the most likely to be docile and accept physicians' prescriptions without question. Furthermore, the physical complaints of older women are often attributed to menopause, psychosomatic causes, or senility (Lewis: 1985; Porcino: 1983).

Since medical education emphasizes acute conditions, many physicians are unfamiliar with the impact of disabilities and the opportunities offered by rehabilitation agencies or have a negative attitude toward rehabilitation. Greenblatt (1989) found that ophthalmologists are themselves unaware of many of the services that exist to help people who are visually impaired or blind. Her study (1991) of people who had recently experienced vision loss found that these individuals are often given a diagnosis with no explanation of the available services or devices that would have enabled them to function independently and to continue working.

A small study by Beckmann and his colleagues (1989) found that most of the women with disabilities they studied had had pelvic examinations and pap smears within the prior 24 months, but their health care providers had not provided information about sexuality. Only one-third of the women felt that their health care providers had enough information about their disabilities to provide information related to sexuality. Nearly half of the women (45.5%) received information about contraception from their health care providers.

Women with disabilities, therefore, face not only the barriers imposed by sex discrimination in the health care system, but also their physicians' lack of knowledge about disabilities and rehabilitation. Compounding these factors are the physical aspects of visiting a physician, including inaccessible examination tables and bathrooms. In addition, women with disabilities are often subject to negative attitudes expressed by staff members who do not know how to accommodate them. According to Nosek (1992), such extreme situations often prevent women with disabilities from seeking out necessary medical care. She also notes that locating an obstetrician/gynecologist who is knowledgeable about the special needs of women with disabilities is extremely difficult.

Given physicians' lack of understanding of the needs and capabilities of women with disabilities, it is not surprising that many women have been advised to have hysterectomies in order to avoid pregnancy. The literature is replete with stories of women who either had medically unnecessary hysterectomies or were advised to have tubal ligations.

Furthermore, women who ask many questions are viewed as "difficult" and as questioning the professionals' competence. Kahan and Gaskill (1978) cite the case of a clinician bemoaning the fact that women have too much information about breast cancer and that "It just stirs them up." Such a statement invalidates a woman's ability to make her own decisions regarding her health care and subjects her to the sole authority of the physician.

Women with disabilities and chronic conditions face a lifetime of visits to physicians and other health care providers. In order to protect their health and obtain information about the best and most recent treatments and products, they must choose their doctors very carefully. Although health maintenance organizations may impose some restrictions on the choice of a physician, in most cases it is possible to "shop around" for a physician. Women should find a physician who takes the time to listen to their complaints, who understands their conditions, and who willingly discusses different treatment approaches and their concomitant risks and benefits. A willingness to respond to a woman's questions and fears, without making her feel that she is taking too much time or is neurotic, is a crucial element in a satisfactory patient-physician relationship.

A woman who feels that her physician does not meet her needs in relation to knowledge about her disability, treatment goals, or communication style should seek another physician. One way to start this process is by asking respected friends and colleagues, preferably those with similar conditions, for referrals. Members of self-help groups or other women's organizations may be good sources. In conducting this search, a woman should phone the prospective physician's office to learn about the physician's office practices, e.g., the physician's knowledge about the woman's condition, who fills in when the physician is not available, physical accessibility of the office and building, times when phone calls are taken, hours of practice, how long it takes to get an appointment, who conducts the examination - the physician or a nurse practitioner. During the first appointment the woman should express her individual needs and concerns in order to discover if the physician's style of practice is amenable. She should make clear what her informational needs are in order to learn if the physician is willing to accommodate them. She should also request copies of all medical reports, including test results, in order to maintain a file of her medical history.

Crewe (1993) refers to a model type of patient-physician relationship for people with disabilities as a consumer-consultant relationship, with greater equality between the participants. Because people who have lived with their disabilities for a period of time become experts not only on the condition itself, but also on their own bodies, they have valuable information to offer to health care providers.

In recent years, some physicians have begun private practices that specialize in women's health. Often these practices include internists, family physicians, and obstetrician/gynecologists with other specialists available for consultation. If these physicians are sensitive to women's needs, they will also have a library or resource center where women may read about their conditions and become knowledgeable about community resources that can help them.

In order to feel that she is obtaining the best possible medical care, a woman should ask questions about the condition, about her specific case, and about alternative treatments and outcomes. The physician may have copies of pertinent articles available to distribute to patients. If no literature is offered, it is a good idea to ask the physician for references on medical studies that support the prescribed treatment method. Physicians who respond that women are unable to understand medical literature feel threatened by questions; those who are confident in their judgment will not hesitate to provide these references. While it is true that not all readers will understand all aspects of every article, most will understand enough to help them with their decisions and to develop a list of additional questions to ask the physician.

Medical school and hospital libraries are often open to the public; if no medical library is available, the local public library or a university library may have medical journals in their collections. Reference librarians at public libraries may obtain copies of articles from other libraries. "Medline," an electronic database with references and abstracts from medical journals, enables users to do subject searches in order to review the pertinent literature on a given condition. "Medline" is available at medical and university libraries, as well as many public libraries.

Not surprisingly, research has shown a significant relationship between disability and depression. A large community based study of individuals with chronic disabilities (Turner and Wood: 1985) found that over a third of the respondents (34.9%) had high scores on a scale that measured depression, indicating that they were clinically depressed. The proportion of individuals with disabilities who were depressed is higher than what would be expected in the general population. Higher proportions of women (40.1%) were depressed than men (28.9%). Higher proportions of respondents who were separated or divorced were depressed than those who were married, with 65% of separated or divorced women depressed compared to 40% of the men. The same study indicates that psychological adaptation to the disability occurs over time, with those whose disabilities had been present the longest least likely to be depressed. Thus, there is empirical evidence that individuals who become disabled go through different psychological stages, usually resulting in acceptance and adaptation.

An important issue for women with disabilities is the sense of lost control over their bodies and their lives. Bodies that do not function properly can disrupt all aspects of life. Planning medications, special diets, attendant care, special transportation, and inquiring about the accessibility of various facilities can all make a woman feel as though she lives in a different world. Brooks and Matson (1987) have described the broad array of coping mechanisms and skills that individuals with multiple sclerosis must develop in order to feel that they have a sense of control over their condition and their lives. They must make decisions about medications and treatment; search for information about their disease; adapt their environment to accommodate their current situation; and take measures to relieve anxiety, all while facing the uncertainty of flares that require different plans. All of these factors affect employment, family life, and relationships outside the family.

Disability and chronic conditions have different impacts depending upon the stage of life at which they occur. When disabilities are congenital, those affected have never experienced life as able-bodied. Nonetheless, their conditions may cause extreme stress within the family and may result in parents spending a great deal of time with the child who is disabled, to the neglect of other children and the parents' own relationship. In cases where the parents' relationship is not strong enough to withstand this stress and divorce results, the child may always feel guilty about the situation. As children with disabilities enter school and become adolescents, they are subject to rejection by both educational institutions and their peers. Obviously, such rejection can be devastating. When young girls begin dating, those with disabilities often find themselves left out, and counselors at schools are not usually trained to help them. The pattern of rejection continues as the girls mature, and women with disabilities are less likely to have romantic partners, whether they be heterosexual or homosexual. In fact, one of the major problems of women with disabilities is loneliness.

Girls learn at a very early age the importance of physical appearance, which becomes a major part of their self-image. Therefore, when a disability causes disfigurement or a change in bodily functioning, self-esteem may be shattered. Women in this situation often fear rejection by their mates, a fear that is not unrealistic. Even in situations where the mates do not reject women with disabilities, the changes that occur in the sexual and family relationships cause a great deal of additional stress. These stress factors evidently contribute to the fact that only a fifth (20.2%) of all women with disabilities are married and living with a spouse. Nearly half (45.4%) live alone (McNeil: 1993).

Women who become disabled or whose chronic conditions occur when they are married and have established families may experience strain within their marriages and families. When women are unable to carry out the roles that they played prior to becoming disabled, their partners or children must fill in the gap. In order to carry out these additional roles, family members must have an understanding of the condition; they must tread a fine line in learning not to do everything for the woman, which may make her feel devalued and guilty. Women whose partners and families become overprotective should draw the line and have frank discussions about their needs, both physical and emotional, and what they can and cannot do. Sexual relations may also be affected, sometimes by the physiological impact of the condition and sometimes due to depression (Rustad: 1984). In strong relationships, where the partner understands the condition and communicates with the woman about both of their needs, the woman benefits from the emotional and instrumental support she receives. As noted above, however, a large portion of women with disabilities live alone and therefore do not receive this support. In addition, women with disabilities are more likely than men to be single heads of families (LaPlante et al.: 1996) and must continue to fulfill this role following the onset of their disability or chronic condition. In cases where conditions flare and abate, emotions may be in constant upheaval, affecting all members of the family.

At midlife, women face a variety of changes that may cause anxiety and depression. Many middle-aged women are facing the "empty nest" syndrome, a situation which may be especially difficult for those who derived their primary identity from being mothers. Normal physical changes, such as aging skin and other symbols of decline in culturally defined physical beauty, contribute to a woman's decreased sense of self-worth. Adding a newly acquired disability to these other major changes in a woman's life may make coping seem an overwhelming task. Support from family, friends, and other women in similar situations may prove invaluable in helping middle-aged women to make the transition from healthy young women to this new stage of life. Williams, writing about women who have reached menopause, notes:

> Women whose self-esteem is intact, whose lives continue to be interesting
> and rewarding, and whose work, whatever its nature, helps them to feel
> that they are making a continuing contribution to the society, are the least
> likely to have negative reactions to the change of life. (1987, 490)

Those women who have acquired disabilities or chronic conditions and who find ways to be productive may also have an easier time adjusting to their new status.

In 1990, there were 31.1 million Americans age 65 or older; of these, 18.6 million were women, and 2.2 million women were age 85 or older. The growth in the older population is expected to continue through the middle of the twenty-first century, because of the aging of the baby boom generation. Women live longer than men, but they also experience higher rates of disabilities. Women 65 years or older are less likely than men to be employed, more likely to be poor, have lower pensions, and less likely to be married (Taeuber and Allen: 1993).

Older women with disabilities and chronic conditions face a different set of circumstances than younger women. Most elders live in the community and nearly a third (30.5%) live alone (U.S. Department of Health and Human Services: 1991). The older a woman gets, the more likely she is to live alone, with over half (54.0%) of all women 85 years or older living alone (U.S. Bureau of the Census: 1990). Older women are often coping with multiple disabilities, including osteoporosis, arthritis, and sensory impairments. For many women, living alone requires a great deal of adaptation, as they had spent many years living with a partner. Members of the oldest group of women have often outlived their friends and relatives, sometimes including their own children. Their support systems are composed of adult offspring, primarily daughters. In cases where daughters do not live in the same area as their mothers, mothers may feel extremely lonely and isolated. Other relatives and friends may be available, but offspring have traditionally been the caregivers for their mothers. Mothers with disabilities who do not have support systems available may have extreme difficulties in coping with their disabilities and experience psychological distress as well. In fact, when applied to a population of elders, the items on a widely used scale designed to measure depression were virtually all significantly associated with physical disability (Berkman et al.: 1986).

How an older woman adapts to recently acquired disabilities depends in part on the coping mechanisms she has developed over a lifetime. Kivnick's (1991) study of elders who ranged from their early 70s to their middle 90s found that those who had developed strong coping mechanisms prevented their disabilities from becoming major handicaps by encapsulating them into one specific area of life and compensating with other behaviors. Those who had more "fragile" personalities were more likely to respond to their disabilities with a sense of despair.

Accepting a disability takes time and the support of others, including family, friends, and women with similar conditions. Sherr Klein, a woman who experienced a severe stroke in mid-life, wrote about her experiences and ultimate acceptance of her new status. Her experience exemplifies how a disability becomes an overriding part of a woman's identity, outweighing her socioeconomic characteristics. However, Sherr Klein's gender and her identity as a feminist enabled her to accept her new status:

> I discover it is easier for me to be a disabled feminist than a disabled
> person. Feminism means loving myself as I am. After three long years,
> I am finally ready to accept myself as permanently, irrevocably disabled...
> (Sherr Klein: 1992, 73)

Accepting the limitations of a disability or chronic condition is not only psychologically liberating, but also makes daily living easier. Zola (1991) discovered that when he finally accepted the label "disabled," he was able to accept the types of assistance he needed in order to make living less of a challenge to his ego. Thus, when he went to airports, he no longer had to prove that he could walk long distances with his crutches but was willing to accept a wheelchair that made his travel easier and enabled him to use his energy for the purpose of his trip. For women with disabilities whose self-esteem is low, reaching this point may be difficult and take time. The willingness to accept assistance, without viewing it as a threat to independence, can help older individuals retain control over their own lives (Kivnick: 1991). The acceptance of realistic limitations and abilities may result in the restoration of self-esteem, the sense of control over life, and pride in achievements for women in all stages of life.

## REHABILITATION FOR WOMEN

Rehabilitation services are available from both public and private providers. The federal government funds rehabilitation services by funneling money to the states. Each state must submit a plan to the federal government indicating how the designated state agency will provide the services required by law. Rehabilitation includes counseling, vocational assessment, job training and placement, provision of assistive technology, training in activities of daily living and homemaking, and transportation services. Women may locate their state's vocational rehabilitation agency by contacting the telephone information operator for the state government.

Originally designed primarily as vocational rehabilitation services, the goals of rehabilitation have been expanded to include the role of homemaker. While learning or re-learning the skills necessary to maintain a home is desirable in order to maintain independence, several studies suggest that women are more likely to receive rehabilitation that trains them to be homemakers, while men receive services that enable them to obtain paid employment (Altman: 1985; Thurber: 1991). Mudrick's study (1987) of recipients of vocational rehabilitation age 50 to 64 years found that women were as likely to receive rehabilitation services as men, but they were less likely to receive job oriented services and more likely to receive physical therapy. A 1993 report by the General Accounting Office cited 1980 data indicating that 29% of women with physical disabilities were rehabilitated as homemakers compared to 8% of men; 83% of men were rehabilitated for competitive employment compared to 67% of women.

Relegating women to the role of homemaker reveals a sexist attitude on the part of the service providers and forces women to remain dependent upon governmental assistance programs for their income. Women should be aware of their options in setting rehabilitation goals. Under federal law, an Individual Written Rehabilitation Program (IWRP) that specifies rehabilitation goals and the services to be provided by the vocational rehabilitation agency must be jointly developed and signed by both the client and the counselor. This means that the woman must agree to both the goals and the means of reaching these goals. Women should ask questions, express interests, and request to see the law when they feel that they are not receiving the services they are entitled to. The IWRP may be amended or modified with reasonable justification and agreement by both parties.

Women who do not know the type of position they are best qualified for should request a functional assessment and a vocational aptitude test. If the vocational rehabilitation agency delays or denies them the opportunity for job training, they should contact the Client Assistance Program. Established under an amendment to the federal Rehabilitation Act (P.L. 98-221), this program informs clients of their rights and all available benefits and assists them in obtaining all remedies due under the law. If this course of action does not result in satisfaction, attorneys who specialize in disability law can provide additional assistance (see Chapter 3, "Laws that Affect Women with Disabilities").

Women with severe disabilities often require assistance with personal care, transportation, and special equipment. Independent living programs enable people with disabilities to continue functioning within the community with assistance. A crucial element of the independent living movement is that consumers have control over the types of services provided. For some, this means living at home, with or without attendant care, and maintaining employment. Attendants assist people with disabilities in activities such as bathing, grooming, dressing, food preparation, and household tasks. Provisions of both Social Security and Medicaid laws have been used to finance the services of attendants. Women with disabilities or chronic conditions may opt to live in group residences, where individuals live under supervision but maintain a degree of responsibility for their own care and maintenance. Independent living programs or centers are sometimes administered by state vocational rehabilitation agencies and sometimes are free-standing organizations administered by individuals with disabilities themselves.

## SEXUALITY AND DISABILITY

(See chapters on specific conditions for information about how sexual functioning is affected by the condition.)

Women find that their disability becomes their primary identity to others, often resulting in rejection by potential sexual partners. The literature repeatedly quotes women with disabilities, whether their disabilities are congenital or acquired later in life, as being viewed by others as asexual. One woman with a mobility impairment noted:

> Once the other person perceives the disability, the switch on the sexual
> circuit breaker often pops off - the connection is broken. "Chemistry" is

over. I have a lifetime of such experiences, and so does every other disabled woman I know. (King: 1993, 72)

Since women in our society are raised to place great value on physical attractiveness, women with disabilities may internalize the view that they are unattractive. Meeting people and seeking potential sexual partners are not only challenging, but may also be assaults on the woman's self-esteem. King notes that she never accepts a date with someone until the other person has seen her walking, to ensure that her disability is made known.

Women who experienced disabilities before adolescence report that their social and sexual encounters occur later and less frequently than those of their peers who were not disabled; they attribute these differences to physical barriers, lack of self-confidence, and negative stereotypes held by peers (Rousso: 1988). The possibility of spasticity during sexual encounters, incontinence, and the use of assistive devices all contribute to the difficulties women with disabilities have in approaching sexual relations with new partners. Parents often counsel their daughters with disabilities to focus on other sources of success, as they fear that they will not be successful in sexual relationships.

Some women with disabilities enter relationships that are less than satisfactory and possibly even abusive, because they fear that no one else will ever want them. Vash (1993) relates the story of how, after becoming paralyzed in her teens, she married a man who convinced her that he was the only one who would want her.

A recent study compared women with disabilities (most had mobility impairments) to women who did not have disabilities (Nosek et al.: 1996). Based on self-administered questionnaires, the study found significant differences between the two groups relative to sexual activity, sexual response, and sexual satisfaction; mean scores for these three variables were higher for the women who did not have disabilities. A fourth component of sexual function, sexual desire, did not appear to be significantly different for the two groups. Severity of disability was not significantly related to sexual activity. The strongest predictor of sexual activity was living with a significant other.

Women who experience disabilities while in an established relationship may avoid resuming sexual activity for fear of failure. Both the woman and her partner may have grave concerns over the new character of their relationship. Mobility impairment, loss of sensation, spasticity, and bowel and bladder incontinence may all seem insurmountable problems at first. Learning new positions for intercourse, additional means of stimulation, and ways to avoid embarrassing leakage problems due to incontinence will relieve the sexual partners of these fears. Sexual counseling, as a couple or in group sessions, can provide invaluable information on these topics. To a great extent, the couple's success at restructuring their sexual relationship depends upon the quality of their relationship prior to the disability; those who had good communications are more likely to be able to discuss their fears and needs openly (Lemon: 1993).

Lesbians with disabilities find that they are marginal to several different movements that are seeking equality for their members: the gay rights movement, the women's movement, and the disability rights movement. The view that heterosexuals have of people with disabilities as being asexual is evidently held for lesbians as well. For example, one lesbian with a disability noted the response she received from a colleague when she declared that she was a lesbian, "How can you be a lesbian if you have no sex?" (Boston Women's Health Book Collective: 1992). Health care providers often ignore the supportive role played by partners of women who are gay and eliminate them from the care of the woman with a disability or chronic condition (Lewis: 1985).

Birth control is another issue that presents special problems for women with disabilities. Women with mobility problems may have difficulty using barrier methods of contraception, such as the diaphragm. Some physical conditions are not amenable to the use of oral contraceptives, as the risks for side effects are increased. The elimination of these methods leaves few alternatives for

16

women with disabilities. One relatively new contraceptive is Norplant, the implantation of a synthetic progesterone that prevents ovulation for as long as five years. Although side effects are minimal, women who take certain antiepileptic drugs are advised against using Norplant (Murphy: 1993). Recently, women have filed suit against the manufacturer of Norplant for pain and scarring associated with its removal.

It is common for both health care providers and rehabilitation professionals to ignore issues of sexuality for women with disabilities. Although the woman's condition itself may cause sexual dysfunction, it is rare to find programs that deal with sexuality, especially for women. Often the programs that do exist are oriented exclusively to the sexual dysfunctions of men. Rehabilitation counselors often ignore sexual preferences, assuming that clients are heterosexual and ignoring lesbian sexuality (Lonsdale: 1990).

Although not all sex therapists are familiar with the needs of women with disabilities, they may prove to be helpful if they are willing to learn about the functional effects of the disability from health care specialists (Cole: 1988) and from the women themselves. Once they are familiar with the woman's mobility limitations, the areas in which she feels stimulation, and other physical factors that affect sexual functioning, the therapist may use traditional history taking and counseling to learn about the woman's psychological attitudes toward sex. With this information, the therapist may help the woman and her partner to learn to feel comfortable with her body and to communicate effectively for a satisfactory sexual relationship.

## PREGNANCY AND CHILDREARING

(See chapters on specific conditions for information about how pregnancy and childrearing are affected by the condition.)

Women with disabilities are often counseled by physicians to be sterilized; those already pregnant are advised to have abortions. This advice is often given by physicians who are unfamiliar with the impact of the disability on the woman's ability to live independently. With most of the disabilities and chronic conditions that are prevalent in women, fertility is unaffected and pregnancy runs a normal course, although extra precautions are sometimes necessary. With some conditions, such as rheumatoid arthritis, pregnancy may actually result in the remission of symptoms, while other conditions, such as epilepsy, may be exacerbated by pregnancy.

Women who are concerned about the possibility of passing their disability on to their children should seek out genetic counseling. Genetic counselors take detailed personal and family health histories to learn about hereditary and environmental causes of disease. They may perform tests to determine if the parents are carriers of genes that cause diseases. Counselors should present information concerning the probability of passing on a given condition but should not be directive in telling prospective parents whether to have children. Providing emotional and educational support for parents is an important function for the counselor, no matter what the couple's decision (Davis: 1978).

In making the decision whether or not to become pregnant, a number of factors should be considered. Among them are the effects of pregnancy on the mother's health; risks to the child; and ability to care for the child. Women who use medications to control symptoms or pain caused by their condition must learn whether these drugs will have deleterious effects on the fetus. Women who experience fatigue as a result of their condition may need to have assistance from a family member or a paid helper. The woman whose condition is exacerbated by fatigue must think about her daily schedule and how it will be affected by pregnancy. The logistics of child care should be discussed with the prospective father and planned in advance to avoid a crisis after the baby arrives. Financial aspects, such as the cost of paid help, should also be considered; some states that provide personal attendants to help the mother do not permit them to perform child care tasks. Mothers who delegate most of their child's care to others may feel left out and unable to bond with their child. Therefore, plans for child care should include the mother to the greatest extent possible.

Women with disabilities feel better about becoming mothers when their partner, family, and friends offer emotional support and help with child care. Roles for taking care of the new baby should be worked out in advance of the birth to avoid the possibility of conflict later. In some cases, fathers may resent the woman with a disability if the additional responsibilities they undertake during pregnancy must be continued after delivery, especially if a flare of the condition occurs. This possibility should be discussed and alternatives planned, so that the father is able to continue with his other activities as well as his share of child care.

Charlifue and colleagues (1992) found that having a child can be overwhelming for women who use wheelchairs. However, the decision to have a child must be a personal one. Campion (1990) suggests that women talk with other women with similar conditions who have children to learn about their experiences with pregnancy and with childrearing.

Once the decision has been made to have a child, finding an obstetrician who is sensitive to the needs of pregnant women with disabilities is the next step, and it may prove to be the most difficult part of the process. Obstetricians are not trained to work with women with disabilities and often have no specialized knowledge of the particular condition involved and its effects on pregnancy. For example, a list of specialists for women with spinal cord injuries included only three physicians in the entire country who specialized in treating pregnant women with this condition. Although it is unlikely that the obstetrician will be a specialist in disabilities, s/he should listen carefully to the woman's description of her condition, her limitations, and her abilities. S/he should also be willing to work with other medical specialists to provide multidisciplinary care.

The physical accessibility of the physician's office may become an issue if the woman needs to use a wheelchair or scooter. Since many obstetrical practices employ several physicians who fill in for each other, it is important that each physician be familiar with the woman's disability and the course of care that has been agreed upon. Other women with disabilities who have children may be the best source of referrals; talking with them may also alleviate the sense of isolation that many pregnant women with disabilities experience. Shaul and her colleagues (1985) discovered that pregnant women with disabilities found the usual informational systems available for pregnant women without disabilities to be very useful for them as well.

A case report (Wasser et al.: 1993) by a woman who has multiple sclerosis and who decided to have a baby illustrates the frustrations that many women with disabilities experience when they decide to have a child. The woman had developed her own methods of self-care to alleviate some of the symptoms of her multiple sclerosis over the course of her disease. When she decided to become pregnant and sought medical care, her physicians refused to acknowledge that her methods were effective and insisted that she first try traditional methods. Not only did her physicians fail to act jointly to coordinate her care, but they failed to provide her with the information she needed to make decisions. She responded by becoming her own de facto case manager, searching for information at medical libraries when her physicians failed to provide sufficient information. Taking this type of assertive action, however, requires a certain type of personality and the education necessary to locate medical literature. This information is becoming more accessible through the availability of Medline, a medical database, at public libraries and over the Internet.

Pregnant women with disabilities may need to be monitored more closely than other women. They may require more frequent visits to the obstetrician, even in the first weeks of pregnancy. Women with diabetes may need to monitor their blood glucose more frequently than usual, as the metabolic changes caused by pregnancy alter glucose processing. Women with spinal cord injuries sometimes need to be hospitalized at the thirty-second week of gestation in order to prepare for labor. In some instances, a cesarean delivery may be necessary.

Teaching the new mother to diaper and bathe her infant may require devising adaptive techniques. Rehabilitation nurses and occupational therapists may work with the maternity nurse and mother to develop these techniques. Hospitals and health maintenance organizations offer classes in child care for prospective parents. Inquiring in advance about the accessibility of the facility and the instructor's knowledge about the effects of the woman's functional disabilities on child care can help the prospective parents find the best program for their specific needs. Since many new mothers with disabilities experience even greater fatigue than mothers without disabilities, it is important to consider labor saving methods.

Modifications to the environment and adaptations to regular equipment to care for babies may be necessary, especially for mothers with mobility impairments. Many women and their families are creative in designing their own baby carriers to attach to wheelchairs and modifying or making changing tables so that a wheelchair fits underneath. Babies learn very quickly to cooperate in ways that accommodate their mothers' needs, by turning their head to find their mother's breast, raising their body for diapering, and holding on for security. A nursing pillow that supports the baby while breastfeeding and a breastpump that is operated by foot enable mothers with mobility impairments to nurse more confidently (see Chapter 2, "VENDORS OF ASSISTIVE DEVICES," page 81).

Couples may find it useful to consult with an occupational therapist, who can make suggestions for adaptive equipment and also suggest safety guidelines. It is important that parents "child proof" their homes while being careful to keep them accessible for the mother. Safety latches for cabinets may be difficult for women with joint disease to open; baby gates must be easy to open for mothers while keeping the toddler safe. Talking with experienced parents may allay many fears and provide a source for adaptive equipment.

Some mothers with disabilities worry about the effect that their disability will have on their children as they grow up. Children of women with disabilities learn at a very early age that they must respond to their mother's verbal admonitions regarding their behavior. In the case of women whose disabilities occur after they have established families, the children may take a long time to adjust to their mother's disabilities and altered lifestyles (Shaul et al.: 1985). Mothers have reported that their disabilities resulted in their children becoming independent, providing support for their mothers, and developing a sensitivity to people who have disabilities. Some mothers, however, are concerned that their children become too independent at an early age and give up some of their childhood in order to help the mothers. Mothers whose disabilities flare worry that their role in their children's lives is inconsistent; these mothers try to provide consistent emotional support as a balance (Thorne: 1990).

Perhaps the greatest barriers to childrearing for women with disabilities are the attitudes expressed by others. As the child begins to socialize with other children and attend school, s/he may be stigmatized by the mother's disability. Parents of other children may be reluctant to let them play at the home of a child whose mother has a disability. Being forthright and explaining the condition and the safety precautions taken for the child's welfare may alleviate some of the fears expressed by other parents. Some mothers deal with these concerns by meeting with teachers before their child starts school, in order to become comfortable with the teacher and vice versa. When parents with disabilities are familiar sights at school activities, everyone benefits. One way to educate children and parents about disabilities is having them participate in exercises where they simulate the conditions in order to learn the limitations imposed by the condition as well as the abilities maintained. Some schools now implement special curricula to teach children about disabilities.

# SELF-HELP FOR WOMEN WITH DISABILITIES

Talking with other women who have had similar experiences can prove to be both cathartic and enlightening. As in any self-help group, women are able to provide each other with suggestions for dealing with common problems, empathy, and shared laughter. A middle-aged woman who experienced a severe stroke discussed the benefits of her experience in DAWN, the DisAbled Women's Network in Canada:

> The DAWN members, typical of disabled women, are mostly un-employed, poor, and living alone. It is like the early days of conscious-ness-raising in the women's movement; sharing painful (and funny) experiences; "clicks" of recognition; swapping tips for coping with social service bureaucracies and choosing the least uncomfortable tampons for prolonged sitting. It is exhilarating to cry and laugh with other women again.

> Here I am not other because everyone is other. It is the sisterhood of disability. The stroke has connected me with women who were not part of my world before - working-class women with little education, women with intellectual and psychiatric disabilities, women with physical "abnormalities" from whom I would have diverted my eyes in polite embarrassment. All women like me. (Sherr Klein: 1992, 73)

Self-help groups enable women with similar problems or conditions to discuss their problems and offer mutual assistance. Self-help groups offer a number of benefits to participants, including learning to develop coping strategies; acquiring a sense of control over life; combating isolation and alienation; and developing information networks. In addition, members of self-help groups often express a sense of increased self-esteem, because they have offered help to other members of the group.

There are local self-help groups for women with disabilities throughout the United States and Canada. To learn about the groups in your area, check the community organizations section in the front of the telephone directory or a directory of local agencies that help individuals with disabilities, found in the reference section of libraries. The United Way information and referral office or a rehabilitation agency may provide referrals to these organizations.

It is often necessary to be creative in establishing self-help groups for women with disabilities. Women who have difficulty traveling because of mobility impairments may have difficulty arranging for transportation to the meeting site. One solution to this problem is to hold meetings by having telephone conference calls (Romness et al.: 1992). While this system may have the disadvantage of not providing face-to-face contact, it does provide the participants with the opportunity to discuss common problems with peers and may eliminate some of the feelings of isolation. Another solution that has become available recently through advanced technology is the use of computer bulletin boards. Using these bulletin boards via a personal computer and a modem, many individuals with shared interests communicate with each other. Individuals with disabilities have a variety of bulletin boards available through generic online services such as CompuServe, America OnLine, and those offered by independent living centers. Individuals who use bulletin boards may exchange information with others who experience the same disabilities or conditions. Individuals have the opportunity to discuss their insights, offer advice, and ask questions; other individuals respond to their questions and comments.

## COMPUTERS AND DISABILITIES

Personal computers (PCs) have opened up a wide variety of opportunities for people who have disabilities or chronic conditions. Used alone, adapted computers enable individuals to perform tasks that would otherwise be inaccessible to them; retaining a job is just one major opportunity that computers offer to people with disabilities. Throughout this book are references to bulletin board services (BBS) operated by agencies as well as Internet resources. Using computers with the Internet, online subscription services, or bulletin board services, individuals are able to communicate with people all over the world. This instant communication provides up-to-the-minute information about new developments and the opportunity to "chat" with individuals in similar situations. Many of these services are free, with the exception of telephone charges or subscription fees for online services.

The reference section of most libraries contains indexes and directories of resources available on the Internet. Look up topics such as disabilities, health, and specific conditions or disabilities. Since new resources become available all the time, sometimes it is necessary to browse various services to obtain up-to-date information. World Wide Web sites and gopher sites provide access to information from government and service agencies, educational institutions, and commercial organizations. One web sites that provides links to information on health and disability is http://www.yahoo.com. Once at this site, a prompt to search results in links to a wealth of information about disabilities. Another strategy for finding resources related to disabilities is to go to a web site of a service organization that provide links to other organizations that provide information in the area of disabilities.

Two sites that offer free access to Medline, a database of articles in medical journals, are http://www.medscape.com and http://www.obgyn.net. A gopher site on the Internet, info.umd.edu, lists Internet resources related to disabilities; choose "educational resources," then "academic resources by topic," then "disability resources." Other sites listed throughout this book provide links to a wide variety of disability resources.

A variety of formats is available to receive and exchange information. When you join a usenet group, you may read messages and respond to them as well as submit your own information and questions. In order to join a usenet group, your host computer must provide access. When you subscribe to a usenet group, you will automatically receive all new messages whenever you log on. If you decide to exchange messages with just one member, you may send mail directly to that individual's e-mail address.

Listserv enables you to receive information by sending a message to an e-mail address stating you would like to subscribe. You may add your own messages which may in turn generate responses from other members of a group. Protocol requires that you then summarize your responses and mail them to all other members of the listserv group.

## CONCLUSION

Women who have come to terms with their disability or chronic condition, who know their rights, and who are able to assert these rights when working with the health care and rehabilitation systems may encounter some frustrations, but ultimately they will gain a feeling that they have taken control of their lives. This important step contributes to improving self-esteem, which in turn enhances social relationships, improves family functioning, and increases the confidence necessary to obtain employment. Setting realistic goals is an important part of this process. Finding health care providers that are knowledgeable and caring, working with rehabilitation professionals, and learning from other women with disabilities are all crucial to maintaining the sense of control which often seems to elude women with disabilities.

References

Altman, Barbara Mandell
1985   "Disabled Women in the Social Structure" pp. 69-76 in Susan E. Browne, Debra Connors, and Nanci Stern (eds.) With the Power of Each Breath Pittsburgh, PA: Cleis Press

Armitage, Karen J., Lawrence J. Schneiderman, and Robert A. Bass
1979   "Response of Physicians to Medical Complaints in Men and Women" JAMA 241(May 18):20:2186-2187

Beckmann, Charles B. et al.
1989   "Gynecologic Health Care of Women with Disabilities" Obstetrics and Gynecology 74(July):1:75-79

Berkman, Lisa F. et al.
1986   "Depressive Symptoms in Relation to Physical Health and Functioning in the Elderly" American Journal of Epidemiology 124:3:372-387

Bonwich, Emily
1985   "Sex Role Attitudes and Role Reorganization in Spinal Cord Injured Women" pp. 56-67 in Mary Jo Deegan and Nancy A. Brooks (eds.) Women and Disability: The Double Handicap New Brunswick, NJ: Transaction

Boston Women's Health Book Collective
1992   The New Our Bodies, Ourselves New York, NY: Simon and Schuster

Brooks, Nancy A. and Ronald R. Matson
1987   "Managing Multiple Sclerosis" Volume 6, pp. 73-106 in Julius A. Roth and Peter Conrad (eds.) Research in the Sociology of Health Care Greenwich, CT: JAI Press Inc.

Campion, Mukti Jain
1990   The Baby Challenge London and New York: Tavistock/Routledge

Charlifue, S.W. et al.
1992   "Sexual Issues of Women With Spinal Cord Injuries" Paraplegia 30:192-199

Cole, Sandra S.
1988   "Women, Sexuality, and Disabilities" Women and Therapy 7:2-3:277-94

Correa, Gena
1975   The Hidden Malpractice: How American Medicine Treats Women as Patients and Professionals New York, NY: William Morrow and Company

Crewe, Nancy M.
1993   "Ageing and Severe Physical Disability" pp.355-361 in Mark Nagler (ed.) Perspectives on Disability Palo Alto, CA: Health Markets Research

Davis, Jessica G.
1978   "Decisions about Reproduction: Genetic Counseling" pp. 33-54 in Malkah T. Notman and Carol C. Nadelson (eds.) The Woman Patient: Medical and Psychological Interfaces New York, NY: Plenum

Deegan, Mary Jo and Nancy A. Brooks (eds.)
1985   Women and Disability: The Double Handicap New Brunswick, NJ: Transaction

DeLozier, James E. and Raymond O. Gagnon

1991   "National Ambulatory Medical Care Survey: 1989 Summary" <u>Advance Data from Vital and Health Statistics</u>  No. 203 Hyattsville, MD: National Center for Health Statistics

Fine, Michelle and Adrienne Asch

1988   <u>Women with Disabilities: Essays in Psychology, Culture and Politics</u> Philadelphia, PA: Temple University Press

1985   "Disabled Women:  Sexism without the Pedestal" pp. 6-22 in Mary Jo Deegan and Nancy A. Brooks (eds.) <u>Women and Disability: The Double Handicap</u> New Brunswick, NJ: Transaction

Greenblatt, Susan L.

1991   "What People with Vision Loss Need to Know"  pp. 7-20 in Susan L. Greenblatt (ed.) <u>Meeting the Needs of People with Vision Loss: A Multidisciplinary Perspective</u>  Lexington, MA: Resources for Rehabilitation

1989   "The Need for Coordinated Care"  pp. 25-38 in Susan L. Greenblatt (ed.) <u>Providing Services for People with Vision Loss: A Multidisciplinary Perspective</u> Lexington, MA:  Resources for Rehabilitation

Howell, Mary C.

1976   "What Medical Schools Teach about Women" <u>New England Journal of Medicine</u> 29(August):304-307

Kahan, Eileen B. and Elizabeth B. Gaskill

1978   "The 'Difficult' Patient: Observations on the Staff-Patient Interaction"  pp. 257-269 in Malkah T. Notman and Carol C. Nadelson (eds.) <u>The Woman Patient: Medical and Psychological Interfaces</u> Volume 1 New York, NY: Plenum

King, Ynestra

1993   "The Other Body: Reflections on Difference, Disability, and Identity Politics" <u>Ms.</u> III(March/April):5:72-75

Kivnick, Helen Q.

1991   "Disability and Psychosocial Development in Old Age"  pp. 92-101 in Robert P. Marinelli and Arthur E. Dell Orto (eds.) <u>The Psychological and Social Impact of Disability</u> New York, NY: Springer Publishing Company

LaPlante, Mitchell P. et al.

1996   "Families with Disabilities in the United States" <u>Disability Statistics Report</u> (8) Washington, DC: U.S. Department of Education, National Institute on Disability and Rehabilitation Research

Lemon, Marilyn

1993   "Sexual Counseling and Spinal Cord Injury" <u>Sexuality and Disability</u> 11:1:73-97

Lewis, Myrna

1985   "Older Women and Health: An Overview" <u>Women and Health</u> 10(Summer/Fall)2/3:1-16

Lonsdale, Susan

1990   <u>Women and Disability</u> New York, NY: St. Martin's Press

McNeil, John M.

1993   <u>Americans with Disabilities 1991-1992</u> Washington DC: U.S. Bureau of the Census  Current Population Reports P70-33

Mudrick, Nancy R.

1987   "Difference in Receipt of Rehabilitation by Impaired Midlife Men and Women" <u>Rehabilitation Psychology</u> 32:1:17-28

Murphy, Eileen

1993   "Norplant: A New Birth Control Option for Women with Disabilities" <u>Resourceful Woman</u> 2(Fall)3:1,5

Nosek, Margaret A.

1992    "Primary Care Issues for Women with Severe Physical Disabilities" <u>Journal of Women's Health</u> 1:4:245-248

Nosek, Margaret A. et al.

1996    "Sexual Functioning among Women with Physical Disabilities" <u>Archives of Physical Medicine and Rehabilitation</u> 77(February):107-115

Porcino, Jane

1983    <u>Growing Older Getting Better: A Handbook for Women in the Second Half of Life</u> Reading, MA: Addison-Wesley Publishing Company

Romness, Sharon, Vicki Bruce, and Catherine Smith-Wilson

1992    "Multiple Sclerosis Telephone Self-Help Support Groups" pp. 220-223 in Alfred H. Katz et al. (eds.) <u>Self-Help: Concepts and Applications</u>  Philadelphia, PA: The Charles Press

Rousso, Harilyn

1988    "Daughters with Disabilities: Defective Women or Minority Women?" pp. 139-171 in Michelle Fine and Adrienne Asch (eds.) <u>Women with Disabilities: Essays in Psychology, Culture and Politics</u> Philadelphia, PA: Temple University Press

Rustad, Lynne C.

1984    "Family Adjustment to Chronic Illness and Disability in Mid-Life" pp. 222-242 in Myron G. Eisenberg, LaFaye C. Sutkin, and Mary A. Jansen (eds.) <u>Chronic Illness and Disability through the Life Span</u>  New York, NY: Springer Publishing Company

Shaul, Susan, Pamela J. Dowling, and Bernice F. Laden

1985    "Like Other Women: Perspectives of Mothers with Physical Disabilities" pp. 133-142 in Mary Jo Deegan and Nancy A. Brooks (eds.) <u>Women and Disability: The Double Handicap</u> New Brunswick, NJ: Transaction

Sherr Klein, Bonnie

1992    "We Are Who You Are" <u>Ms.</u> III(November/December):3:70-74

Taeuber, Cynthia M. and Jessie Allen

1993    "Women in Our Aging Society: The Demographic Outlook" pp. 11-45 in Jessie Allen and Allen Pifer (eds.) <u>Women on the Front Lines: Meeting the Challenge of an Aging America</u> Washington, DC: Urban Institute Press

Thorne, Sally E.

1990    "Mothers with Chronic Illness: A Predicament of Social Construction" <u>Health Care for Women International</u> 11:209-221

Thurber, Shari L.

1991    "Women and Rehabilitation" pp. 32-38 in Robert P. Marinelli and Arthur E. Dell Orto (eds.) <u>The Psychological and Social Impact of Disability</u> New York, NY: Springer Publishing Company

Turner, R. Jay and D. William Wood

1985    "Depression and Disability: The Stress Process in a Chronically Strained Population" <u>Research in Community and Mental Health</u> 5:77-109

U.S. Bureau of the Census

1990    "Marital Status and Living Arrangements March 1989" <u>Current Population Reports</u>, Series P-20 No. 445(June) cited in U.S. Senate Special Committee on Aging <u>Aging in America: Trends and Projections 1991 Edition</u>

U.S. Department of Health and Human Services

1991    <u>Aging in America: Trends and Projections</u> Washington, DC: U.S. Department of Health and Human Services, DHHS Publication No. (FCoA) 91-28001

24

U.S. General Accounting Office

1993  <u>Vocational Rehabilitation: Evidence for Federal Program's Effectiveness is Mixed</u> GAO/PEMD-93-19

Vash, Carolyn L.

1993  "Sexuality Ascending" <u>Sexuality and Disability</u> 11:2:149-157

Wasser, Andrea M., Carrie L. Killoran, and Sarah S. Bansen

1993  "Pregnancy and Disability" <u>AWHONN's Clinical Issues</u> 4:2:328-337

Williams, Juanita

1987  <u>Psychology of Women: Behavior in a Biosocial Context</u> New York, NY: W. W. Norton

Zola, Irving Kenneth

1991  "Bringing Our Bodies and Ourselves Back In:  Reflections on a Past, Present, and Future 'Medical Sociology'" <u>Journal of Health and Social Behavior</u> 32(March):1-16

# ORGANIZATIONS

Alliance of Genetic Support Groups
35 Wisconsin Circle, Suite 440
Chevy Chase, MD 20815
(800) 336-4363                      (301) 652-5553                      FAX (301) 654-0171
e-mail: alliance@capaccess.org      http://medhelp.org/www/agsg.htm

Provides education and services to families and individuals affected by genetic disorders.  Membership, individuals, $25.00; organizations, $50.00; includes monthly news bulletin, "ALERT."

American Association of Sex Educators, Counselors and Therapists (AASECT)
PO Box 238
Mount Vernon, IA 52314-0238

A membership organization for professionals who counsel individuals with sexual dysfunctions.  AASECT will provide lists of its members in a local geographical area upon receipt of a self-addressed, stamped, business size envelope.

American Medical Women's Association (AMWA)
801 North Fairfax Street, Suite 400
Alexandria, VA 22314-1757
(703) 838-0500                      FAX (703) 549-3864

A professional membership organization for women in the field of medicine.  Addresses health issues specific to women and promotes equal status for women within the field of medicine.  Publishes booklets to guide women who are contemplating a career in medicine and a directory of members.  Some branches offer referrals to local women physicians.

American Self-Help Clearinghouse
St. Clares-Riverside Medical Center
Pocono Road
Denville, NJ 07834
(201) 625-7101                      (201) 625-9053 (TT)                FAX (201) 625-8848
e-mail: ASHC@bc.cybernex.net        http://www.cmhc.com/selfhelp/

A clearinghouse that makes referrals to national, state, or local self-help groups.  Publishes a variety of materials for professionals and consumers who would like to start self-help groups, including "Ideas and Considerations for Starting a Self-Help Mutual Aid Group," "Suggestions on Locating a Meeting Place," and "Suggested Techniques for Recruiting Group Members."  Semi-annual newsletter, "Network."  Free

Canadian Rehabilitation Council for the Disabled (CRCD)
45 Sheppard Avenue East, Suite 801
Toronto, Ontario M2N 5W9 Canada
(416) 250-7490 (V/TT)               FAX (416) 229-1371

A federation of regional and provincial groups that serve people with disabilities in Canada. Operates an information service and publishes a newsletter, "Access," and "Rehabilitation Digest," a quarterly journal with news about rehabilitation in Canada.

Center for Research on Women with Disabilities (CROWD)
Baylor College of Medicine
3440 Richmond Avenue, Suite B
Houston, TX 77046
(713) 960-0505 (V/TT)          FAX (713) 961-3555
e-mail: mnosek@bcm.tmc.edu          http://www.bcm.tmc.edu/crowd/

A federally funded center that conducts research and develops and distributes information on the health and independence of women with disabilities. Research areas include sexuality, relationships, general health, reproductive health, and abuse. Executive Summary of a four year "National Study on Women with Disabilities" is available; $20.00.

Combined Health Information Database (CHID)
Ovid Technologies, Attn: CHID Database
333 7th Avenue
New York, NY 10001
(800) 950-2035          (212) 563-3006

A federally sponsored database for service providers and consumers; includes bibliographic citations and abstracts from journals, reports, and education programs. Special files on eye health, cancer patient education, cancer prevention and control, and diabetes. Available at many libraries, or services may be purchased for use on a personal computer.

Commission on Accreditation of Rehabilitation Facilities (CARF)
4891 East Grant Road
Tucson, AZ 85712
(520) 325-1044 (V/TT)          FAX (520) 318-1129          http://www.carf.org

Conducts site evaluations and accredits organizations that provide rehabilitation. Publishes the "Directory of Accredited Organizations," $45.00 plus $5.50 shipping and handling.

Department of Veterans Affairs (VA)
(800) 827-1000

This nationwide toll-free number connects veterans with the VA regional office in their vicinity. The VA has funded eight Comprehensive Women's Centers around the country to provide medical and mental health care; however, all VA Medical Centers have clinics for women veterans. Disability need not be service connected in order to receive services.

National Association of Sibling Programs (NASP)
Sibling Support Project
Children's Hospital and Medical Center
PO Box 5371
Seattle, WA 98105
(206) 368-4911                          FAX (206) 368-4816
e-mail: dmeyer@chmc.org


Maintains a database of sibling programs across the U.S. Includes programs for young siblings of children with developmental disabilities and chronic illness and for adult siblings.


National Black Women's Health Project
1211 Connecticut Avenue, NW, Suite 310
Washington, DC 20036
(202) 835-0117                          FAX (202) 833-8790
e-mail: NBWHPDC@aol.com


Advocates on behalf of black women and promotes physical and mental well-being through self-help, technical assistance, and training. Membership, $25.00, includes quarterly newsletter, "Vital Signs."


National Council on Disability (NCD)
1331 F Street, NW, 10th Floor
Washington, DC 20004
(202) 272-2004              (202) 272-2074 (TT)              FAX (202) 272-2022
http://www.ncd.gov


An independent federal agency mandated to study and make recommendations about public policy for people with disabilities. Holds regular meetings and hearings in various locations around the country. Publishes newsletter, "Focus," available in standard print, large print, or on audiocassette. Free


National Health Information Center (NHIC)
PO Box 1133
Washington, DC 20013-1133
(800) 336-4797              In MD, (301) 565-4167              FAX (301) 984-4256
e-mail: nhicinfo@health.org              http://nhic-nt.health.org


Maintains a database of health-related organizations and a library. Provides referrals related to health issues for both professionals and consumers. Publications enable individuals to locate information and resources in the federal government. Free publications list.


National Institute on Disability and Rehabilitation Research (NIDRR)
U.S. Department of Education
400 Maryland Avenue, SW
Washington, DC 20202
(202) 205-8134              (202) 205-8198 (TT)              FAX (202) 205-8515
http://www.ed.gov/offices/OSERS/NIDRR

A federal agency that supports research into various aspects of disability and rehabilitation, including demographic analyses, social science research, and the development of assistive devices. Grant programs are announced in the "Federal Register" (see "PUBLICATIONS AND TAPES" section below) or may be obtained directly from NIDRR.

National Lesbian and Gay Health Association
1407 S Street, NW
Washington, DC 20009
(202) 939-7880                    FAX (202) 234-1467

This network of lesbian and gay community health centers, health educators, researchers, and service providers provides education, advocacy, and technical assistance to its members. Membership, $60.00, includes quarterly newsletter, "The Health Advocate."

National Library of Medicine (NLM)
8600 Rockville Pike
Building 38, Room 2S-10
Bethesda, MD 20894
(800) 272-4787                    (301) 496-6095                    http://www.nlm.nih.gov

Operates MEDLINE, a computerized database of articles in major medical journals from around the world. Users may search for a specific health related topic and receive citations and abstracts of articles. Available directly through NLM and through the Internet, subscription services, and at most medical, public, and university libraries.

National Library Service for the Blind and Physically Handicapped (NLS)
1291 Taylor Street, NW
Washington, DC 20542
(800) 424-8567 or (800) 424-8572 (Reference Section)
(800) 424-9100 (to receive application)
(202) 707-5100                    FAX (202) 707-0712
telnet marvel.loc.gov (log in as marvel, select Library of Congress Online Systems, select connect to LOCIS, then select "Braille and Audio" for a catalogue of braille and tape publications)

Provides services to all adults and children with print handicaps, including those who cannot hold a book or turn pages, through a network of regional libraries. Provides publications in braille, on audiocassette and flexible disc, and the machines to play them. Some NLS libraries also distribute large print books. A health professional must certify that the individual is unable to hold a book or turn pages; has blurred or double vision; extreme weakness or excessive fatigue; or other physical limitations which prevent her from reading standard print. All services from NLS are free.

National Rehabilitation Association (NRA)
633 South Washington Street
Alexandria, VA 22314
(703) 836-0850                    (703) 836-0849 (TT)                    FAX (703) 836-0848
http://www.allware.com/rehab/

A professional membership organization for rehabilitation professionals and independent living center affiliates. Includes special divisions for independent living, counseling, job placement, etc. Legislative alerts appear on NRA's home page on the World Wide Web. Regular membership, $85.00, includes "Journal of Rehabilitation" and newsletter, "Contemporary Rehab," associate member, $57.00 (journal not included); student, $10.00.

National Rehabilitation Information Center (NARIC)
8455 Colesville Road, Suite 935
Silver Spring, MD 20910-3319
(800) 346-2742                          (301) 588-9284                          (301) 495-5626 (TT)
FAX (301) 587-1967                  e-mail: naric@capaccess.org
http://www.naric.com/naric

A federally funded center that responds to telephone and mail inquiries about disabilities and support services. Maintains "REHABDATA," a database with publications and research references. Some NARIC publications are available on the World Wide Web site.

National Research and Training Center on Families of Adults with Disabilities
Through the Looking Glass
2198 Sixth Street, #100
Berkeley, CA 94710-2204
(800) 644-2666                          (510) 848-1112                          FAX (510) 848-4445
e-mail: tlg@lookingglass.org      http://www.lookingglass.org

A federally funded research and training center that conducts research on the needs of parents with disabilities. Conducts research on special equipment and techniques of caring for babies. Maintains a national network of parents with disabilities, their families, researchers, and service providers. Publishes "Parenting with a Disability," a newsletter with information about the center's activities, publications in the field, and practical information for parents. Available in standard print and large print. Free

National Self-Help Clearinghouse
Graduate School and University Center/CUNY
25 West 43rd Street, Room 620
New York, NY 10036
(212) 642-2944

Makes referrals to local self-help groups and self-help group clearinghouses throughout the nation. Publishes quarterly newsletter, "The Self-Help Reporter," $10.00.

National Women's Health Network
514 10th Street, NW, Suite 400
Washington, DC 20004
(202) 347-1140                          FAX (202) 347-1168

A coalition of consumers, health care providers, and researchers who work to provide up-to-date information about women's health issues and to improve women's ability to make informed decisions about their health care. Maintains a clearinghouse to provide information on a wide variety of disorders and conditions that affect women. Membership, $25.00, includes bimonthly newsletter "Network News."

National Women's Health Resource Center
2425 L Street, NW, 3rd Floor
Washington, DC 20037
(202) 293-6045                    FAX (202) 293-7256

Develops programs and clinical services to meet women's health needs; sponsors conferences; and provides information to encourage women to be active participants in their own health care decisions. Maintains a database on women's health issues and provides responses to telephone inquiries about specific health issues with referrals, resources, and general information. Membership, individuals, $25.00; organizations, $75.00; includes bimonthly newsletter, "National Women's Health Report."

Office of Research on Women's Health (ORWH)
National Institutes of Health (NIH)
Building 1, Room 201
Bethesda, MD 20892
(301) 402-1770                    FAX (301) 402-1798
http://www.nih.gov/od/odp/whi/

Established in 1990, this organization monitors NIH policy with the goal of promoting research into diseases that are prevalent in women, affect only women, have different effects on women than on men, or have different risk factors or interventions for women. ORWH works to ensure that women are represented in NIH sponsored research and to develop opportunities for recruitment, retention, and advancement of women in biomedical careers. Coordinates the Women's Health Initiative (WHI), a research project that sponsors clinical trials, observational studies, and community prevention strategies. A randomized controlled clinical trial of about 65,000 postmenopausal women age 50 to 79 is investigating the role of diet in the prevention of breast and colon cancer and coronary heart disease; the effects of estrogen replacement on prevention of osteoporotic fractures and heart disease; and how calcium and vitamin D supplements affect prevention of osteoporotic fractures and colon cancer. Forty Clinical Centers have been established to study postmenopausal women across the country, including ten specifically recruiting African-American and Hispanic women, Asian-Americans/Pacific Islanders, and Native Americans. The Community Prevention Study will evaluate how to encourage women to adopt healthful behaviors.

Older Women's League (OWL)
666 11th Street, NW, Suite 700
Washington, DC 20001
(800) 825-3695                    (202) 783-6686                    FAX (202) 638-2356
(202) 783-6689 (OWL Powerline; taped weekly information on legislative issues affecting midlife and older women)

Advocates on behalf of older women in areas such as health, housing, and financial affairs. Publishes research papers, model bills for state legislative action, books, and videotapes. Membership, $25.00, includes bimonthly newsletter, "The Owl Observer."

Research and Training Center on Independent Living (RTC/IL)
University of Kansas
4089 Dole Building
Lawrence, KS 66045
(913) 864-4095 (V/TT)            FAX (913) 864-5063
e-mail: rtcil@kuhub.cc.ukans.Edu     http://www.lsi.ukans.edu/rtcil/rtcbroc.htm

A federally funded center that conducts research and training on the variables that affect independent living.  Publications catalogue, free.

Resources for Rehabilitation
33 Bedford Street, Suite 19A
Lexington, MA 02173
(617) 862-6455            FAX (617) 861-7517

A private nonprofit organization that provides training and information to professionals who serve people with disabilities and to the public.  Conducts custom designed training programs, program evaluations, and needs assessments.

Rural Institute on Disabilities
52 Corbin Hall
University of Montana
Missoula, MT 59812
(800) 732-0323            (406) 243-5467            (406) 243-4200 (TT)
FAX (406) 243-2349

A federally funded center that conducts research and training on issues that affect service delivery of rehabilitation in rural areas.  Maintains a directory of rural disability services throughout the country.  Publishes a quarterly newsletter, "Rural Exchange."   Free

Sex Information and Education Council of Canada (SIECCAN)
850 Coxwell Avenue
East York, Ontario M4C 5R1 Canada
(416) 466-5304            FAX (416) 778-0785

Provides information and education about sexuality through conferences, publications, and a network of members who  serve as referral resources.  Membership, individuals, Canada, $35.00; U.S., $45.00; organizations, Canada, $50.00; U.S., $60.00 (Canadian funds); includes "Canadian Journal of Human Sexuality," quarterly, and the SIECCANewsletter."

Sexuality Information and Education Council of the United States (SIECUS)
130 West 42nd Street, Suite 350
New York, NY 10036-7802
(212) 819-9770            FAX (212) 819-9776
e-mail: siecus@siecus.org     http://www.siecus.org

Provides information and education about sexuality through publications, database, library, symposia, and advocacy. Membership, individuals, $75.00; organizations, $135.00; includes bimonthly journal, "SIECUS Report." Publications catalogue, free.

Society for Disability Studies (SDS)
c/o David Pfeiffer
Department of Public Management
Suffolk University
8 Ashburton Place
Boston, MA 02108-2770
(617) 523-3429                          (617) 523-3682 (TT)

Membership organization of practitioners, clinicians, and social scientists interested in the study of issues related to disability. Holds an annual meeting. Membership dues vary by income level.

Society for the Scientific Study of Sex
PO Box 208
Mount Vernon, IA 52314-0208
(319) 895-8407                          FAX (319) 895-6230

A multidisciplinary society of professionals who conduct research on sex; includes a special interest group on disability. Membership, $110.00, includes "Journal of Sex Research," nonmembers subscription, individuals $63.00; institutions, $100.00.

TASH: The Association for Persons with Severe Handicaps
29 West Susquehanna Avenue, Suite 210
Baltimore, MD 21204
(410) 828-8274                 (410) 828-1306 (TT)           FAX (410) 828-6706

A national advocacy organization that disseminates information to improve the education and increase the independence of individuals with severe disabilities. Holds an annual conference. Regular membership, $72.00; parent/student/paraprofessional membership, $49.00; includes "Journal of the Association for Persons with Severe Handicaps," quarterly, and the "TASH Newsletter."

United Way of America (UW)
701 North Fairfax Street
Alexandria, VA 22314-2045
(800) 892-2757                 (703) 836-7100                FAX (703) 683-7840
http://www.unitedway.org

United Way/Centraide Canada
56 Sparks Street, Suite 404
Ottawa, Ontario K1P 5A9 Canada
(613) 236-7041                 FAX (613) 236-3087

An umbrella organization of local human service organizations. National offices in the U.S. and Canada direct callers to the local United Way, which in turn will provide referrals to local service agencies.

VISIBLE
PO Box 91304
Santa Barbara, CA 93101
(805) 966-7796

Advocates on behalf of lesbians and all women over age 60. Newsletter published three times per year; sliding fee scale.

Well Spouse Foundation
610 Lexington Avenue, Suite 814
New York, NY 10022
(800) 838-0879                    (212) 644-1241                    FAX (212) 644-1338
e-mail: wellspouse@aol.com

A network of support groups that provide emotional support to husbands, wives and partners of people who are chronically ill. Membership, U.S., $20.00; foreign, $25.00; professional membership, $50.00; includes bimonthly newsletter, "Mainstay." Publishes pamphlets discussing "Guilt," "Anger," "Isolation," and "Looking Ahead." $1.50 each; $5.00 per set.

Women's Initiative (WIN)
American Association of Retired Persons (AARP)
601 E Street, NW
Washington, DC 20049
(800) 424-3410                    (202) 434-2277                    http://www.aarp.org

Advocates to improve the status of older women, including women with disabilities. Deals with health, economic, long term care, and social issues. Each area and state AARP office has a contact person for the WIN program. Publishes fact sheets and semi-annual newsletter, "AARP WIN Women's Initiative Network." Free

World Institute on Disability (WID)
510 Sixteenth Street, Suite 100
Oakland, CA 94612
(510) 763-4100                    (510) 208-9493 (TT)                    FAX (510) 763-4109
e-mail: wid@wid.org              http://www.igc.org/wid

A public policy center founded and operated by individuals with disabilities, WID conducts research, public education, and training; it also develops model programs related to disability. It deals with issues such as personal assistance, public transportation, employment, and access to health care. WID's Research and Training Center on Public Policy in Independent Living (PPIL) is a federally funded center that studies personal assistance services, federal independent living initiatives, and community integration issues. Operates the WIDNet electronic bulletin board system, which includes databases of laws, regulations, journal articles, and research studies.

ABLED
12211 Fondren, Suite 703
Houston, TX 77035
(713) 726-1132                    FAX (713) 726-1132                    e-mail: ablepubl@aol.com

A newsletter that provides advice from physicians, attorneys, and other who work with women with disabilities; articles written by women with disabilities about their experiences; and research results. Free.  Also available on audiocassette for $2.00 from Taping for the Blind, 3935 Essex Lane, Houston, TX 77027. (713) 622-2767

Across Borders: Women with Disabilities Working Together
by Diane Drieger, Irene Feika, and Eileen Giron Batres (eds.)
gynergy books
PO Box 2023
Charlottetown, Prince Edward Island C1A 7N7 Canada
(902) 566-5750                    FAX (902) 566-4473
e-mail: booksales@gynergy.com

This anthology written by women with disabilities discusses their personal lives and political activism in both developed and developing countries.  U.S., $14.95; Canada, $16.95; plus $3.00 shipping and handling; Canadian funds.

Adaptive Parenting Equipment: Idea Book I
Through the Looking Glass
2198 Sixth Street, #100
Berkeley, CA 94710-2204
(800) 644-2666                    (510) 848-1112                    FAX (510) 848-4445
e-mail: tlg@lookingglass.org          http://www.lookingglass.org

A book that describes 50 products to help women with disabilities diaper, bathe, dress, feed, and play with their babies.  Individuals, $10.00; organizations, $25.00.

Beyond Rage: Mastering Unavoidable Health Changes
by JoAnn LeMaistre
Alpine Guild
PO Box 4846
Dillon, CO 80435
(800) 869-9559                    FAX (970) 262-9378

Written by a woman with multiple sclerosis, this book describes the emotional responses to health changes due to physical disabilities, chronic illness, and aging.  Print, $24.95; abridged version on audiocassette, $12.95.

Building Community: A Manual Exploring Issues of Women and Disability
Educational Equity Concepts
114 East 32nd Street, Suite 701
New York, NY 10016
(212) 725-1803                    FAX (212) 725-0947

A collection of readings and activities that explore the relationship between gender and disability bias. Available in standard print, braille, and audiocassette. Individuals, $15.00; institutions, $25.00; plus 15% shipping and handling.

Dictionary of Rehabilitation
by Myron G. Eisenberg
Springer Publishing Company
536 Broadway
New York, NY 10012
(212) 431-4370                    FAX (212) 941-7842

This book defines the core terms used in the rehabilitation field. $43.95 plus $3.50 shipping and handling.

Disability and Motherhood
Fanlight Productions
47 Halifax Street
Boston, MA 02130
(800) 937-4113                    (617) 542-0980                    FAX (617) 524-8838
e-mail: fanlight@tiac.net        http://www.fanlight.com

This videotape portrays the childbearing and childrearing experiences of three women with disabilities. 25 minutes. $149.00

Disability in America: Toward a National Agenda for Prevention
National Academy Press
2101 Constitution Avenue, NW
Lockbox 285
Washington, DC 20055
(800) 624-6242                    (202) 334-3313                    FAX (202) 334-2451

The report of a panel of experts, this book examines the magnitude of disability in the U.S., recommends a model to prevent disabilities, and makes a series of policy recommendations. $29.95 plus $4.00 shipping and handling.

Disability in the United States: A Portrait from National Data
by Susan Thompson-Hoffman and Inez Fitzgerald-Storck (eds.)
Springer Publishing Company
536 Broadway
New York, NY 10012
(212) 431-4370                    FAX (212) 941-7842

This collection of articles based on data collected from a variety of federal agencies analyzes the relationship between a wide variety of demographic characteristics and disability with implications for future policy and research. $38.95 plus $3.50 shipping and handling.

Disability Studies Quarterly
c/o David Pfeiffer
Department of Public Management
Suffolk University
8 Ashburton Place
Boston, MA 02108-2770
(617) 523-3429                    (617) 523-3682 (TT)

A quarterly journal with reports on recent research findings, upcoming meetings, and grant solicitations. Reviews of books and audio-visual materials. Available in standard print, audiocassette, e-mail, and computer disk (PC). Individuals, $35.00; institutions, $45.00.

The Disabled Women's Theatre Project
Women Make Movies
462 Broadway, Suite 500 E
New York, NY 10013
(212) 925-0606              FAX (212) 925-2052              e-mail: orders@wmm.com

Written and performed by women with disabilities, this videotape uses dance, drama, and comedy to portray the absurd, joyous, and painful experiences that the women have encountered. 60 minutes. Purchase, $295.00; rental for three days, $75.00; plus $15.00 shipping and handling.

Double the Trouble, Twice the Fun
Women Make Movies
462 Broadway, Suite 500 E
New York, NY 10013
(212) 925-0606              FAX (212) 925-2052              e-mail: orders@wmm.com

In this videotape, interviews are conducted with both lesbians and gays, dispelling the myth that people with disabilities are asexual. 25 minutes. Purchase, $50.00; rental for three days, $75.00; plus $15.00 shipping and handling.

Dykes, Disability & Stuff
PO Box 8773
Madison, WI 53708

This newsletter advocates for access for lesbians with disabilities including access to lesbian culture. Available in print, large print, braille, audiocassette, DOS diskette, and modem transfer. Sliding scale rates: individual, $10.00 to $25.00; organization, $25.00 to $50.00.

Enabling Romance: A Guide to Love, Sex, and Relationships for the Disabled
by Ken Kroll and Erica Levy Klein
Woodbine House
6510 Bells Mill Road
Bethesda, MD 20817
(800) 843-7323                    (301) 897-3570                    FAX (301) 897-5838
e-mail: woodbine85@aol.com

Written by a man who has a disability and his wife who does not, this book provides examples of how people with a variety of disabilities have established fulfilling relationships. $15.95 plus $4.00 shipping and handling.

Encyclopedia of Disability and Rehabilitation
by Arthur E. Dell Orto and Robert P. Marinelli (eds.)
Macmillan Library Reference
866 Third Avenue, 2nd Floor
New York, NY 10022
(800) 223-2336                    (800) 223-1244

Written by a variety of experts in the field of disability, this reference book includes articles ranging from AIDS to stroke, advocacy to wheelchairs, and aging to work. $105.00 plus $4.00 shipping and handling.

Federal Register
New Orders, Superintendent of Documents
PO Box 371954
Pittsburgh, PA 15250-7954
(202) 512-1800                    FAX (202) 512-2250
telnet federal.bbs.gpo.gov (Port 3001) BBS (202) 512-1661
e-mail: gpoaccess@gpo.gov            http://www.access.gpo.gov/su_docs/aces/desc004.html

A federal publication printed every weekday with notices of all regulations and legal notices issued by federal agencies. Domestic subscriptions, $494.00 annually for second class mailing of paper format; $433.00 annually for microfiche. Available at federal depository libraries. Also available on the Internet at no charge.

Frank Talk
by JoAnn LeMaistre
Alpine Guild
PO Box 4846
Dillon, CO 80435
(800) 869-9559                    FAX (970) 262-9378

In this videotape, individuals share their concerns about living with chronic illness and discuss coping strategies. 30 minutes. $39.95

Handicapped Moms - Mothers of Invention
Mary Free Bed Hospital and Rehabilitation Center
235 Wealthy Street, SE
Grand Rapids, MI 49503
(616) 242-0429                    (616) 454-3939

In this videotape, two women with disabilities discuss the methods they have devised to raise their children and the barriers they have had to overcome. 9 minutes. Purchase, $165.00; rental for 10 working days, $35.00.

Helping You Helps Me
by Karen Hill
Canadian Council on Social Development
441, MacLaren, 4th Floor
Ottawa, Ontario K2P 2H3 Canada
(613) 236-8977                FAX (613) 236-2750                e-mail: council@ccsd.ca
http://www.achilles.net/~council/

This book provides practical information on starting and maintaining a self-help group. $8.00, Canadian funds.

Imprinting Our Image: An International Anthology by Women with Disabilities
Diane Driedger and Susan Gray (eds.)
gynergy books
PO Box 2023
Charlottetown, Prince Edward Island C1A 7N7 Canada
(902) 566-5750                FAX (902) 566-4473
e-mail: booksales@gynergy.com

This collection of essays written by women with disabilities discusses their changing roles in the family and the community in both developed and underdeveloped countries. $12.95 plus $3.00 shipping and handling, Canadian funds.

Independent Living
Equal Opportunity Publications
1160 East Jericho Turnpike, Suite 200
Huntington, NY 11743
(516) 421-9421

A magazine that addresses the needs of individuals with disabilities in everyday life, including careers and health care issues. Articles written by professionals and consumers. Published seven times a year, including an annual "Resource Directory & Buyers' Guide." $18.00

Intimate Resources for Persons with Disabilities
Sureen Publishing
Box 23102
124 Welland Avenue
St. Catharines, Ontario L2R 7P6 Canada
FAX (905) 688-2935

This directory lists resources for information, products, and services in areas such as sexuality, incontinence, sex aids, and newsletters and specialty magazines. $12.95, Canadian funds.

It's Okay
Sureen Publishing
Box 23102
St. Catharines, Ontario L2R 7P6 Canada
FAX (905) 688-2935

Written by people with disabilities, this quarterly magazine emphasizes love and sexuality. U.S., $23.95; Canada, $23.95, Canadian funds.

Journal of Disability Policy Studies
Department of Rehabilitation Education and Research
346 North West Avenue
Fayetteville, AR 72701
(501) 575-3656 (V/TT)           FAX (501) 575-3253

A journal, published twice a year, with articles related to legislative policy and regulatory matters as well as articles from a range of academic disciplines. U.S., $24.00; foreign, $29.00.

Journal of Rehabilitation
National Rehabilitation Association (NRA)
633 South Washington Street
Alexandria, VA 22314
(703) 836-0850           (703) 836-0849 (TT)           FAX (703) 836-0848
http://www.allware.com/rehab/

A quarterly journal with articles related to the provision of rehabilitation services and psychological responses to disabilities, plus book reviews. Subscription, U.S., $50.00; Canada, $60.00; foreign, $75.00.

Journal of Rehabilitation Research and Development (JRRD)
Scientific and Technical Publications Section
Rehabilitation Research and Development Service
103 South Gay Street, 5th Floor
Baltimore, MD 21202
(410) 962-1800

A quarterly journal that includes articles on rehabilitation, sensory aids, gerontology, and disabling conditions. Annual supplements provide research progress reports. Clinical supplements report on specific topics. Free

Journal of Women and Aging
Haworth Press
10 Alice Street
Binghamton, NY 13904
(800) 342-9678            (607) 722-5857            FAX (800) 895-0582
e-mail: getinfo@haworth.com

A multidisciplinary quarterly journal that publishes articles dealing with psychosocial practice, theory and research. Individuals, $40.00; organizations, $90.00; libraries, $175.00.

Journal of Women's Health
Mary Ann Liebert, Inc., Publishers
2 Madison Avenue
Larchmont, NY 10538
(800) 654-3237            (914) 834-3100            FAX (914) 834-1388

A bimonthly journal that publishes articles dealing with the conditions and diseases that are prevalent in women. Individuals, $61.00, plus $12.00 shipping and handling; institutions, $152.00, plus $15.00 shipping and handling.

Kaleidoscope
United Disability Services
326 Locust Street
Akron, OH 44302
(330) 762-9755            (330) 379-3349 (TT)            FAX (330) 762-0912

A magazine that explores disability through articles of fiction, poetry, and fine art. Contributions by individuals with disabilities and individuals without disabilities. Two issues per year. Individuals, $9.00; institutions, $14.00; Canada, add $5.00; foreign, add $8.00.

Mainstream
2973 Beach Street
San Diego, CA 92102
(619) 234-3138            http://www.mainstream-mag.com

A magazine with articles, information about products, and a calendar of events. Ten issues per year. One year, $24.00; two years, $44.00.

Making Disability
by Paul Higgins
Charles C. Thomas Publisher
2600 South First Street
Springfield, IL 62794
(800) 258-8980                    (217) 789-8980                    FAX (217) 789-9130
e-mail: books@ccthomas.com        http://www.ccthomas.com

Written by a sociologist, this book examines disability as a social phenomenon rather than a defect. It discusses the depiction of disability, experiencing disability, serving individuals with disabilities, and developing disability policy. Hardcover, $51.95; softcover, $30.95; plus $5.50 shipping and handling.

The Me in the Mirror
by Connie Panzarino
Seal Press
3131 Western Avenue, Suite 410
Seattle, WA 98121
(800) 754-0271                    (206) 283-7844                    FAX (206) 285-9410
e-mail: sealprss@scn.org          http://www.seanet.com/~sealpress/

Written by a woman who was born with spinal muscular atrophy III, a disease that has resulted in severe mobility impairment, this book provides details about her education, work, familial relationships, and romantic relationships, including her eventual turn to lesbianism. $12.95 plus 16.5% shipping and handling.

Mothers with Disabilities: An Introduction to Issues
Health Resource Center for Women with Disabilities
Rehabilitation Institute of Chicago
345 East Superior Street, Room 683
Chicago, IL 60611
(312) 908-7997                    (312) 908-8523 (TT)              e-mail: jpsparkle@aol.com

In this videotape, women with mobility impairments discuss their pregnancies, their experiences with the adoption process, and their coping strategies. A psychologist analyzes the overriding issues that the women have presented. 20 minutes. $10.00

Mother-to-Be: A Guide to Pregnancy and Birth For Women with Disabilities
by Judith Rogers and Molleen Matsumura
Demos Vermande
386 Park Avenue South, Suite 201
New York, NY 10016
(800) 532-8663                    (212) 683-0072                  FAX (212) 683-0118

This book describes the pregnancy and childbirth experiences of 36 women with a wide variety of disabilities. Suggests practical solutions for the special concerns of women with disabilities during pregnancy and those of their partners, families, and health care providers. Includes a list of resources, glossary, and bibliography. $24.95 plus $4.00 shipping and handling.

The National Guide to Funding for Women and Girls
The Foundation Center
79 Fifth Avenue, Department KK
New York, NY 10003-3076
(800) 424-9836                    (212) 620-4230                    FAX (212) 807-3677

This directory provides information about foundations and corporations that fund programs for women and girls.  $95.00 plus $4.50 shipping and handling.

The New Ourselves Growing Older
by Paula B. Doress-Worters and Diana Laskin Siegal
Simon and Schuster
200 Old Tappan Road
Old Tappan, NJ 07675
(800) 223-2348                    e-mail: ss cust serv@prenhall.com
http://www.simonsays.com

This book provides information and resources for midlife and older women.  Topics include aging, sexuality, disabilities, health care, employment, housing, and finances.  $18.00 plus $3.00 shipping and handling.

No Pity: People with Disabilities Forging a New Civil Rights Movement
by Joseph P. Shapiro
Random House
400 Hahn Road
Westminster, MD 21157
(800) 293-2665                    (410) 848-1900                    FAX (410) 386-7013
http://www.randomhouse.com

This book describes the evolution of the disability rights movement and profiles its leaders.  $15.00 plus $4.00 shipping and handling.

Past Due: A Story of Disability, Pregnancy, and Birth
by Anne Finger
Seal Press
3131 Western Avenue, Suite 410
Seattle, WA 98121
(800) 754-0271                    (206) 283-7844                    FAX (206) 285-9410
e-mail: sealprss@scn.org          http://www.seanet.com/ ~ sealpress/

In this autobiographical book, a woman who was disabled by polio analyzes the issues pertinent to disability and pregnancy.  $10.95 plus 16.5% shipping and handling.

Peer Counseling for Seniors
Senior Health and Peer Counseling
2125 Arizona Avenue
Santa Monica, CA 90404-1398
(310) 828-1243                    FAX (310) 453-8485

This trainers' guide is designed to help service providers prepare volunteers to conduct peer counseling sessions for older adults. Includes a manual, audiocassettes, and handouts, $375.00. Videotapes on effective training and supervision are also available.

Positive Images
Women Make Movies
462 Broadway, Suite 500 E
New York, NY 10013
(212) 925-0606                    FAX (212) 925-2052                    e-mail: orders@wmm.com

In this videotape, three women (one blind, one deaf, and one with a spinal cord injury) discuss their lives at home, at work, and with family and friends. 58 minutes. Purchase, $295.00; rental for three days, $75.00; plus $15.00 shipping and handling.

Ragged EDGE
Advocado Press
Box 145
Louisville, KY 40201
(501) 894-9492                    FAX (501) 899-9562                    e-mail: rgarr@iglou.com
http://www.iglou.com/why/edge

This magazine reports on disability issues from the perspective of disability rights activists. Individuals, $17.50; institutions, $35.00; Canada, $42.00. Also available online at the World Wide Web site.

Report on Disability Programs
Business Publishers
951 Pershing Drive
Silver Spring, MD 20910
(800) 274-0122                    (301) 587-6300                    FAX (301) 585-9075

A biweekly newsletter with information on policies promulgated by federal agencies, laws, and funding sources. $297.00

Reproductive Issues for Persons with Physical Disabilities
by Florence P. Haseltine, Sandra S. Cole, and David B. Gray (eds.)
Brookes Publishing Company
PO Box 10624
Baltimore, MD 21285-9945
(800) 638-3775                    e-mail: custserv@p.brookes.com

This book provides an overview of sexuality, disability, and reproductive issues across the lifespan for individuals with disabilities including multiple sclerosis and spinal cord injury. Includes academic articles as well as personal narratives written by individuals with disabilities. $34.00

Resourceful Woman
Health Resource Center for Women with Disabilities
Rehabilitation Institute of Chicago
345 East Superior Street, Room 683
Chicago, IL 60611
(312) 908-7997                    (312) 908-8523 (TT)                    e-mail: jpsparkle@aol.com

A newsletter dealing with the broad range of issues that affect women with disabilities. Includes a regular column "Resourceful Parenting," which answers readers' questions. Free (contribution requested).

The Self-Help Sourcebook
American Self-Help Clearinghouse
St. Clares-Riverside Medical Center
Pocono Road
Denville, NJ 07834
(201) 625-7101                    (201) 625-9053 (TT)          FAX (201) 625-8848
e-mail: ASHC@bc.cybernex.net     http://www.cmhc.com/selfhelp/

Provides information on national and model self-help groups, online mutual help groups and networks, and self-help clearinghouses. Includes chapters on starting self-help groups. $9.00

The Self-Help Way: Mutual Aid and Health
by Jean-Marie Romeder
Canadian Council on Social Development
441, MacLaren, 4th Floor
Ottawa, Ontario K2P 2H3 Canada
(613) 236-8977                    FAX (613) 236-2750                    e-mail: council@ccsd.ca
www.achilles.net/~council/

This book discusses the dynamics of self-help and describes the growth of the self-help movement. Hardcover, $30.00; softcover, $20.00; Canadian funds.

Sexual Concerns When Illness or Disability Strikes
by Carol L. Sandowski
Charles C. Thomas Publisher
2600 South First Street
Springfield, IL 62794
(800) 258-8980                    (217) 789-8980                    FAX (217) 789-9130
e-mail: books@ccthomas.com       http://www.ccthomas.com

Written by a social worker who is a certified sex counselor, this book discusses sexuality and issues of self-esteem that arise with illness or disability. $35.95 plus $5.50 shipping and handling.

Sexuality and Disability
Human Sciences Press
233 Spring Street
New York, NY 10013-1578
(800) 221-9369                    (212) 620-8000                    FAX (212) 807-1047

A quarterly journal with articles on the medical and rehabilitation aspects of sexuality for individuals who have experienced a disability. Individuals, U.S. $49.00; foreign, $57.00; institutions, U.S., $185.00; foreign, $215.00.

Sexuality and Disability
Sexuality Information and Education Council of the United States (SIECUS)
130 West 42nd Street, Suite 350
New York, NY 10036-7802
(212) 819-9770                    FAX (212) 819-9776
e-mail: siecus@siecus.org        http://www.siecus.org

This annotated bibliography lists general books, books for professionals, curricula, journals and newsletters, teaching aids, databases, and organizations that provide information about sexuality for individuals with disabilities. $2.00

Strategies for Maintaining a Support Group
by Pearl R. Paulson
Women's Educational Equity Act Publishing Center
55 Chapel Street, Suite 200
Newton, MA 02158
(800) 225-3088                    (617) 969-7100                    FAX (617) 332-4318

This book helps support groups for women with disabilities work through difficulties, maintain open communications, and delegate responsibilities. $9.50 plus $3.50 shipping and handling.

Table Manners: A Guide to the Pelvic Examination for Disabled Women and Health Care Providers
by Susan Ferreyra and Katrine Hughes
Planned Parenthood Alameda/San Francisco
815 Eddy Street
San Francisco, CA 94109
(415) 441-7858                    FAX (415) 776-1449

Written by two women with disabilities, this booklet suggests alternative positions for pelvic examinations; discusses bowel and bladder concerns, spasticity, and hypersensitivity; and describes transfer methods for getting on the examination table. $1.50 plus $3.25 shipping and handling.

Us and Them
Fanlight Productions
47 Halifax Street
Boston, MA 02130
(800) 937-4113                    (617) 542-0980                    FAX (617) 524-8838
e-mail: fanlight@tiac.net        http://www.fanlight.com

This videotape is about relationships between people who have disabilities and those who do not. 32 minutes, black and white. Purchase, $69.00; rental for one day, $50.00; plus $9.00 shipping charge.

We Are Not Alone: Learning to Live with Chronic Illness
by Sefra Kobrin Pitzele
Workman Publishing
708 Broadway
New York, NY 10003
(800) 722-7202                    (212) 254-5900

Written by a woman with lupus, this book offers practical advice for coping with chronic diseases and maintaining relationships. It also provides practical suggestions for independent living. $10.95 plus $3.00 shipping and handling.

With the Power of Each Breath
Susan E. Browne, Debra Connors, and Nanci Stern
Cleis Press
PO Box 8933
Pittsburgh, PA 15221
(800) 780-2279                    (412) 937-1555                    FAX (412) 937-1567
e-mail: pghcleis@aol.com

This collection of articles written by women with a variety of disabilities describes their experiences, their emotions, and societal reactions. $10.95 plus 15% shipping and handling.

With Wings: An Anthology of Literature by and about Women with Disabilities
by Marsha Saxton and Florence Howe (eds.)
The Feminist Press of the City University of New York
311 East 94th Street
New York, NY 10128
(212) 360-5794                    FAX (212) 348-1241

In this collection of articles, women with a variety of disabilities and from varied backgrounds discuss their conditions, their feelings, society's reactions, and how they have worked to empower themselves. $14.95 plus $4.00 shipping and handling.

Women and Health
Haworth Press
10 Alice Street
Binghamton, NY 13904
(800) 342-9678                    (607) 722-5857                    FAX (800) 895-0582
e-mail: getinfo@haworth.com

A multidisciplinary quarterly journal that deals with all phases of health care, including disability, rehabilitation, and chronic illness. Individuals, $45.00; institutions, $190.00; libraries, $250.00.

Women and Their Doctors
by John M. Smith
Grove/Atlantic

Written by a gynecologist, this book discusses the abuse of women by the medical system, medical problems experienced by women, when certain procedures are appropriate, and how to select the right gynecologist. Out of print.

Women's Health Issues
Elsevier Science Publishing Company
655 Avenue of the Americas
New York, NY 10010
(212) 633-3750

A multidisciplinary quarterly journal with articles related to the medical, social, and legal aspects of health care delivery. Individuals, $42.00; institutions, $84.00.

Women with Physical Disabilities
by Danuta M. Krotoski, Margaret A. Nosek, and Margaret A. Turk (eds.)
Brookes Publishing Company
PO Box 10624
Baltimore, MD 21285-9945
(800) 638-3775                         e-mail: custserv@p.brookes.com

This collection of articles addresses the special issues that women with disabilities face, including self-concept, dating and relationships, sexuality, pregnancy and motherhood, and bowel and bladder control. $42.00

You Are Not Your Illness
by Linda Noble Topf
Simon and Schuster
200 Old Tappan Road
Old Tappan, NJ 07675
(800) 223-2348                         e-mail: ss cust serv@prenhall.com
http://www.simonsays.com

In this book, the author, who has multiple sclerosis, shares her personal perspectives on living with chronic illness. She describes a step-by-step process for dealing with loss and maintaining feelings of self-worth. $12.00 plus $3.00 shipping and handling.

# Chapter 2

# COPING WITH DAILY ACTIVITIES

Women in our society carry out a variety of roles and responsibilities; they are mothers, career women, and caregivers for sick or disabled partners or parents. For women with disabilities, these activities may become a challenge. Although the number of products to help people with disabilities live independently has increased dramatically in recent years, especially with the advent of the personal computer, the everyday tasks performed by women with disabilities are often more time consuming than they are for healthy women. And while increasing numbers of women have entered the workforce, it is well known that women are still responsible for the major portion of household activities, even when partners are available to provide assistance. After a discussion of the effects of disabilities on the family, the sections that follow provide information about carrying out basic everyday activities, providing care for others with disabilities, working with a disability, housing and environmental adaptations, and recreation and travel.

## HOW DISABILITIES AND CHRONIC CONDITIONS AFFECT THE FAMILY

Diagnosis of a disability or chronic condition in a family member can cause disruption in the healthiest of families. Coping with a crisis situation puts strain on any relationship; coping with the inevitability of a permanent change causes strain between marital partners and places great stress upon children. Stress may be related to providing adequate health care, financial concerns, disruption of familiar patterns of everyday living and work, and sexual relations.

Children in the family are often not told the details of the situation, as parents do not want to frighten them. Without information, however, their imaginations may picture a situation far worse than reality. During the initial crisis, when their mother is in the hospital, the children are often deprived not only of her company but also of their father's, who is tending to the mother's emotional and physical needs (Rustad: 1984).

It is crucial that family members understand the nature of the condition and its effects on daily functioning. Holding realistic expectations for what the affected family member can and cannot do contributes to the individual's ability to cope with the situation. Being overly protective and trying to do everything for the affected family member may result in diminished self-esteem and independence. On the other hand, expecting the individual to carry out activities that are unrealistic or implying that the limitations are "only in the head" creates a great deal of additional stress. People with disabilities and chronic conditions often express the fear of being a burden on family members; when their relatives suggest that they can accomplish tasks that are physically impossible for them, the affected individuals will be reluctant to ask for assistance at any time.

Following the onset of a disability or chronic condition, all family members must be prepared for role changes and accommodations. The woman who has been affected may find that she can no longer carry out the roles in the family that she was accustomed to. For example, if she is no longer able to drive, she will not be able to transport children to activities or go grocery shopping on her own. Her partner or spouse will need to take on additional roles. Children who are old enough should be encouraged to take on some additional household responsibilities. When it is financially feasible, hiring household help can alleviate some of the burdens placed on family members. Some families may qualify for homemaker services provided by government agencies or voluntary organizations.

Often the assistance of a social worker or a psychologist is necessary to help the family restructuring that takes place following the development of a disability or chronic condition. The emotional needs of the spouse or partner must also be considered. Since the spouse or partner has the additional role of providing emotional and physical support for the individual who has developed a disability or chronic condition, he or she will likely need support also. Self-help groups of other caregivers in similar situations may prove helpful. Hulnick and Hulnick (1989) suggest that counselors can help family members "reframe" the context of the situation so that they respond positively, learn and grow from the new situation, and empower themselves to make choices. Local and state governments, private agencies that provide case management services, and voluntary organizations that are dedicated to one disease or disability often have programs to help family members as well as the individuals with disabilities and chronic conditions.

## CARING FOR OTHERS WITH DISABILITIES

Women provide most of the "informal" care required by their parents and spouses. Although many caregivers are middle-aged women, as the population lives longer women 65 years or older may simultaneously be providing care for their spouses and for their elderly parents (usually mothers) who may be 85 years or older. These older caregivers themselves may also be experiencing the effects of chronic health problems and disabilities.

Women caring for partners who have disabilities not only face the physical demands such caregiving entails but the emotional issues that spring from changes in the relationship. Cohen, whose husband has multiple sclerosis, describes the "dire straits" in which she and their children lived until her husband moved to a nursing home. Despite participation in multiple sclerosis support groups and well spouse groups, she felt that she experienced a conspiracy of silence about the realities of family caregiving that kept her ignorant of caregiving options. This situation led her to comment:

> Well spouses often feel weak, ineffective, and perhaps ashamed and guilt ridden. Our belief systems are threatened. We're forced, or feel we're forced, to go against our beliefs, our habits, our life-styles, and our expectations. (1996, 120)

The extreme stresses she endured caused Cohen to question her role in the marriage, "I don't know to what extent I am still a wife, to what extent I want to be" (1996, 81).

Sons are far less likely than daughters to provide care for their parents. When parents have no daughters, it is usually the daughters-in-law who provide the care, not the sons. When sons do provide assistance, it is often in the domain of financial management. Daughters, accepting their roles as nurturers, may make excuses for their brothers' failure to help by asserting that men's work is their primary function. All the while, these daughters may be juggling their own families and work schedules to provide care for parents (Aronson: 1992).

Adding the role of caregiver to an already overburdened lifestyle may result in great stress. Often the caregiver must take time away from her employment outside the home in order to carry out the necessary caregiving tasks. These tasks include providing transportation, arranging for medical appointments, shopping and other household tasks, and supervising medication. In some instances, helping relatives with disabilities includes helping them with the basic tasks of living, such as bathing, dressing, and eating.

The emotional and physical burden of providing these tasks for an older relative while taking care of her family of procreation often causes conflict for a woman. Children may find that their mother is not available as often as they would like or when she is available, she is too tired to participate in the usual family activities. The sheer quantity of caregiving indicates why caregivers are "women in the middle;" Brody (1990) found that three-quarters of daughters provided care every single day. Furthermore, the older the caregiver (and therefore her mother), the greater number of hours per week she spent providing care (Brody: 1981).

A recent study (Richards and Shewchuk: 1996) found that most caregivers of individuals with spinal cord injuries were women, usually wives or mothers. Not only was a majority of this sample clinically depressed, but their positive affect decreased between six months and one year following discharge from the hospital. Not surprisingly, caregivers for individuals who were quadriplegics had higher levels of emotional distress than caregivers of individuals who were paraplegics. While the stress for caregivers of paraplegics declined over time, the stress for caregivers of quadriplegics increased, suggesting that the severity of the condition plays a role in the caregivers' emotional problems. Caregivers spent a substantial part of their day carrying out the tasks associated with caring for the person with spinal cord injury.

Caregiving for a parent may result in feelings of anger, guilt, and depression. Psychological conflicts that existed between mothers and daughters may be rekindled; problems that already existed between spouses may intensify as a result of the additional demands on time and emotions. When caregivers enter into a relationship with the relative's health care provider, additional conflicts may ensue, as the caregiver and the health care provider may hold an opinion contrary to the relative's (Haug: 1994).

As difficult as this situation is for healthy women, women who have disabilities or chronic conditions may feel that they are neglecting their parents if they do not help with the provision of care and services. While they may hold unrealistic expectations for themselves, they may feel guilty for not being able to devote time or energy to their parents. In such situations, locating a case manager for the parent may be the most useful solution. Some case managers are in private practice, while others may be located at publicly funded agencies on aging. Case managers will evaluate the person's needs, recommend appropriate services, and follow up to ensure that the services are being provided.

To relieve the burden on family members, many state departments on aging fund programs that provide assistance to elders living at home who need additional care. Financial assistance is also available. Employment of a home health aide alleviates some of the burdens placed on the family caregiver. Respite care programs, which may include activities outside the home for the care recipient or home health aides to assist with grooming and other daily activities, enable caregivers time to take care of their own needs. In addition, adult day care programs provide transportation and activities for elders with disabilities. Both of these programs may be available from agencies that serve elders, hospitals, or visiting nurse associations. Another option that may prove useful to the woman who finds herself in the role of caregiver is a support group of family members in similar situations. Many of the national voluntary organizations that are dedicated to a single disease or disability sponsor these support groups.

Employers, recognizing the growing needs of their employees in the area of elder care, have begun to provide assistance as well. Flexible time schedules, information and referral services, and on-site adult day care are a few of the programs that are now available at places of employment.

The federal Family and Medical Leave Act of 1993 (P.L. 103-3) enables eligible employees to take unpaid leave from work to care for sick relatives without forfeiting their jobs or their benefits (see Chapter 3, "Laws that Affect Women with Disabilities" for a more detailed description of this act).

References

Aronson, Jane
1992    "Women's Sense of Responsibility for the Care of Older People: 'But Who Else is Going to Do It?'" Gender and Society 6(March):1:8-29

Brody, Elaine M.

1990 <u>Women in the Middle: Their Parent Care Years</u> New York, NY: Springer Publishing Company

1981 "'Women in the Middle' and Family Help to Older People" <u>The Gerontologist</u> 21:5:471-479

Cohen, Marion Deutsche

1996 <u>dirty details: the days and nights of a well spouse</u> Philadelphia, PA: Temple University Press

Haug, Marie R.

1994 "Elderly Patients, Caregivers, and Physicians: Theory and Research on Health Care Triads" <u>Journal of Health and Social Behavior</u> 35(March):1-12

Hulnick, Mary R. and H. Ronald Hulnick

1989 "Life's Challenges: Curse or Opportunity? Counseling Families of Persons with Disabilities" <u>Journal of Counseling and Development</u> 68(November/December):166-170

Richards, J. Scott and Richard Shewchuk

1996 "Caregivers of Persons with Spinal Cord Injury: A Longitudinal Investigation" <u>Research Update</u> Spain Rehabilitation Center, University of Alabama at Birmingham, September

Rustad, Lynne C.

1984 "Family Adjustment to Chronic Illness and Disability in Mid-Life" pp. 222-242 in Myron G. Eisenberg, LaFaye C. Sutkin, and Mary A. Jansen (eds.) <u>Chronic Illness and Disability through the Life Span</u> New York, NY: Springer Publishing Company

# ORGANIZATIONS

Children of Aging Parents (CAPS)
Woodbourne Office Campus, Suite 302A
1609 Woodbourne
Levittown, PA 19057
(215) 945-6900

Helps caregivers find the appropriate care and support for elders as well as for themselves. Sponsors a network of support groups for caregivers. Publishes a variety of training and resource materials for support groups, a national directory of geriatric case managers, and a newsletter, "CAPSule." Membership, U.S., individuals, $15.00; professionals and organizations, $25.00; outside U.S., individuals, $20.00; professionals and organizations, $30.00.

Eldercare Locator
National Association of Area Agencies on Aging (NAAAA)
(800) 677-1116                     (202) 296-8130

A nationwide telephone information and referral service that provides callers with the phone number for an information and referral service in their local area, which in turn provides the name of a local agency that can help with their specific needs. Free

National Family Caregivers Association
9621 East Bexhill Drive
Kensington, MD 20895-3104
(301) 942-6430                     FAX (301) 942-2302

A membership organization for individuals who provide care for others at any stage of their lives or with any disease or disability. Maintains an information clearinghouse and a network of individuals who would like to provide and receive support from others in similar situations. Membership, individuals, $15.00; professionals, $30.00; nonprofit organizations, $50.00; group medical practices, home health agencies, etc., $100.00; hospitals and corporate providers, $200.00.

National Research and Training Center on Families of Adults with Disabilities
Through the Looking Glass
2198 Sixth Street, Suite 100
Berkeley, CA 94710-2204
(800) 644-2666                     (510) 848-1112                     FAX (510) 848-4445
e-mail: tlg@lookingglass.org       http://www.lookingglass.org

A federally funded center that conducts research on the needs of parents with disabilities. Conducts research on special equipment and techniques of caring for babies. Maintains a national network of parents with disabilities, their families, researchers, and service providers. Publishes "Parenting with a Disability," a newsletter with information about the center's activities, publications in the field, and practical suggestions for parents. Available in standard print and large print. Free

Well Spouse Foundation
610 Lexington Avenue, Suite 814
New York, NY 10022
(800) 838-0879                    (212) 644-1241                    FAX (212) 644-1338
e-mail: wellspouse@aol.com

A network of support groups that provide emotional support to husbands, wives and partners of people who are chronically ill.   Membership, U.S., $20.00; foreign, $25.00; professional membership, $50.00; includes bimonthly newsletter, "Mainstay."  Publishes pamphlets discussing "Guilt," "Anger," "Isolation," and "Looking Ahead."  $1.50 each; $5.00 per set.

Work and Family Clearinghouse
Women's Bureau
U.S. Department of Labor
200 Constitution Avenue, NW, Room S 3306
Washington, DC 20210
(800) 827-5335                    (202) 219-4486
http://www.dol.gov/dol/wb/

Provides information to employers on financial assistance, public-private partnerships, and information services related to eldercare.

# PUBLICATIONS AND TAPES

Answers: The Magazine for Adult Children of Aging Parents
201 Tamal Vista Boulevard
Corte Madera, CA 94925-9800
(415) 924-4737

A magazine that covers a wide range of issues related to caregiving for elders. Topics covered include living arrangements, nutrition, insurance, legal matters, and helpful resources. Also included is a feature that responds to readers' questions. Six issues per year. U.S., $15.00; Canada, $27.00.

The Caregiver's Guide: Helping Elderly Relatives Cope with Health and Safety Problems
by Caroline Rob and Janet Reynolds
Houghton Mifflin Company
181 Ballardvale Street
Wilmington, MA 01887
(800) 225-3362                    FAX (800) 634-7568

This book covers a wide range of health problems, including cancer, pain, pneumonia, skin disease, digestive problems, and sleep disorders. $13.95 plus $3.00 shipping and handling.

dirty details, the days and nights of a well spouse
by Marion Deutsche Cohen
Temple University Press
1601 North Broad Street
Philadelphia, PA 19122-6099
(800) 447-1656                    FAX (215) 204-4719
e-mail: tempress@astro.ocis.temple.edu

A frank, personal account, written by a woman whose husband has multiple sclerosis, this book describes her caregiving experiences. Hardcover, $49.95; softcover, $16.95; plus $4.00 shipping and handling.

Families and Aging: Dilemmas and Decisions
Extension
Oregon State University
Ballard Extension Hall 125
Corvallis, OR 97331-3604
(503) 737-4131

An educational game that helps participants understand family dynamics by playing a variety of roles and expressing their concerns through discussions with other players. $20.00

Families and Health
National Council on Family Relations (NCFR)
3989 Central Avenue, NE, Suite 550
Minneapolis, MN 55421
(612) 781-9331                    FAX (612) 781-9348
e-mail: ncfr398@aol.com

This videotape discusses how families cope with chronic illness and disability, how they interact with health care professionals, and how the caregiver's management of stress affects the entire family. 90 minutes. $49.95

Family Caregivers
Films for the Humanities & Sciences
PO Box 2053
Princeton, NJ 08543-2053
(800) 257-5126                    FAX (609) 275-3767

This videotape offers suggestions for dealing with the stresses of caregiving and profiles the Well Spouse Foundation (see "ORGANIZATIONS" section above). 30 minutes. $89.95 plus $5.75 shipping and handling.

Family Caregiver's Guide
by Joan Ellen Foyder
National Stroke Association
96 Inverness Drive East, Suite I
Englewood, Colorado 80112-5112
(800) 787-6537              (303) 649-9299              FAX (303) 649-1328
e-mail: info@stroke.org

A book that provides practical information and emotional support for caregivers. Includes sources for medical supplies and equipment and assistive devices. $6.00 plus $3.00 shipping and handling.

A Guide to Helping Elderly Relatives Near and Far
by Pam Erickson and Gordon Wolfe
National Stroke Association
96 Inverness Drive East, Suite I
Englewood, Colorado 80112-5112
(800) 787-6537              (303) 649-9299              FAX (303) 649-1328
e-mail: info@stroke.org

An audiocassette that emphasizes communication and teamwork to help elders remain independent; written by a nurse and a social worker. $19.95 plus $3.00 shipping and handling.

Helping Yourself Help Others: A Book for Caregivers
by Rosalynn Carter with Susan K. Golant
Random House
400 Hahn Road, PO Box 100
Westminster, MD 21157
(800) 293-2665          (410) 848-1900          FAX (410) 386-7013
http://www.randomhouse.com

This book focuses on family caregivers, offering suggestions for everyday problems such as physical and emotional needs, isolation, burnout, and dealing with professional caregivers. Lists of organizations, books, and resources included. $20.00

Hiring Home Caregivers: The Family Guide to In-Home Eldercare
by D. Helen Susik
American Source Books
PO Box 1094
San Luis Obispo, CA 93406-1094
(800) 246-7228          (805) 543-5911          FAX (805) 543-4093
e-mail: 74133.303@compuserv.com

This book provides practical information for elders and family members for directly hiring, supervising, and paying home caregivers. Included are sample forms for recruiting, interviewing, and checking references of potential caregivers as well as employment agreements and suggestions for supervision. $11.95 plus $4.00 shipping and handling.

How to Help Children Through a Parent's Serious Illness
by Kathleen McCue with Ron Bonn
St. Martin's Press
175 Fifth Avenue
New York, NY 10010
(800) 221-7945

This book presents practical guidelines to help parents explain their illness to children of different ages, how to understand the children's reactions, and how to seek professional help. Includes a chapter on chronic illness. $18.95

Life Services Planning for the Elderly and Persons with Disabilities
Commission on Mental and Physical Disability Law
American Bar Association
740 15th Street, NW, 9th Floor
Washington, DC 20005-1009
(202) 662-1570          (202) 662-1012 (TT)          FAX (202) 662-1032
e-mail: cmpdl@abanet.org          http://www.abanet.org

This three book series provides guidance for individuals, families, and service providers in estate, financial, health care, and government benefits planning. $20.00 plus $3.95 shipping and handling.

Long Distance Caregiving: A Survival Guide for Far Away Caregivers
by Angela Heath
American Source Books
PO Box 1094
San Luis Obispo, CA 93406-1094
(800) 246-7228                (805) 543-5911                FAX (805) 543-4093
e-mail: 74133.303@compuserv.com

This book helps caregivers who do not live in the same area as their relatives locate assistance, deal with emergencies, and arrange financial and legal affairs. $12.95 plus $4.00 shipping and handling.

The Other Victim - Caregivers Share Their Coping Strategies
by Alan Drattell
Seven Locks Press
PO Box 25689
Santa Ana, CA 92799
(800) 354-5348

This book is a collection of personal accounts of nine caregivers of individuals with multiple sclerosis. Includes resource list of organizations. $17.95 plus $4.00 shipping and handling.

Share the Care
by Cappy Capossela and Sheila Warnock
Simon and Schuster
200 Old Tappan Road
Old Tappan, NJ 07675
(800) 223-2348                e-mail: ss cust serv@prenhall.com
http://www.simonsays.com

This book provides guidelines for sharing responsibilities for the care of a person who is seriously ill. $13.00 plus $3.00 shipping and handling.

Someone Who Cares
Terra Nova Films
9848 South Winchester Avenue
Chicago, IL 60643
(800) 779-8491                (773) 881-8491                FAX (773) 881-3368
e-mail: info@terranova.org

This videotape shows how frail elders can maintain their independence with the assistance of home care workers. Includes workbook, "A Guide to Hiring an In-home Caregiver." Purchase, $145.00; rental, $45.00; plus $9.00 shipping and handling.

Unending Work and Care: Managing Chronic Illness at Home
by Juliet M. Corbin and Anselm Strauss
Jossey-Bass Inc.
350 Sansome Street
San Francisco, CA 94104
(415) 433-1767                    http://josseybass.com

This book analyzes the issues that affect the lives of individuals with chronic illness and their family members.  Describes physical and emotional needs; the role of health care personnel; and the means to manage chronic illness effectively.  $45.00 plus $7.50 shipping and handling.

The Women's Legal Defense Fund's Guide to Using the Family and Medical Leave Act: Questions and Answers
Women's Legal Defense Fund
1875 Connecticut Avenue, NW, Suite 710
Washington, DC 20009
(202) 986-2600                    FAX (202) 986-2539

This booklet answers the most frequently asked questions about the law.  $10.00

## WORKING WITH A DISABILITY

Women with disabilities are less likely to be in the workforce than men with disabilities or than healthy men or women. Individuals in higher paying, white collar positions are more likely to retain their jobs after disability. Because women in general and women with disabilities in particular have had fewer opportunities for educational achievement than men, they are less likely than men to be employed following disability. Just over half (52.0%) of all Americans with disabilities age 21 to 64 years are employed; however, only 45.2% of women with disabilities are employed compared to 59.1% of men (McNeil: 1993). Women with work disabilities are nearly three times as likely to be unemployed as women without disabilities (U.S. Department of Labor Women's Bureau: 1992). Thus, while women in the general population are seeking to break through the "glass ceiling" in order to achieve equity with men, women with disabilities are not even at an equal status with their healthy female peers.

Because many women had been full-time homemakers or had low paying, part-time positions prior to their disability, they are unlikely to have private disability insurance or workers' compensation. Most women with disabilities (82.5%) receive one or more types of financial assistance from the government: food stamps, cash assistance, or household assistance (McNeil: 1993).

Many women with disabilities and chronic conditions experience extreme fatigue, which makes them feel unproductive. These women often feel it appears that they are shirking their responsibilities when their physical condition requires that they live at a much slower pace than what they were accustomed to (Hillyer: 1993). Changes in physical abilities may require that women adopt different definitions of productivity without feeling guilty. Women who previously held full-time positions while managing a house and raising children may find it necessary to hire household help, cut back on working hours, and require that family members carry out household chores. Other options that can help eliminate fatigue are flexi-time schedules, job sharing with another person to cut down on hours, and performing work at home to eliminate travel time. Working at home full-time, however, can lead to an increased sense of isolation, a problem that is prevalent among women with disabilities.

One woman who had experienced a severe stroke found that slowing down was not all bad:

> Being forced to slow down is not all negative. The rhythm of my life has changed dramatically. Before, it was governed by the calendar and the clock. Now I follow the natural pace of my body. The tasks of everyday living take me much longer. I have become patient, as have those around me. I have to ration my limited energy and choose carefully who I see and what I do. I have no time to waste on bullshit, but I do have time to smell the flowers. I cherish my solitude, and enjoy the fullness of the company of intimate friends and family. (Sherr Klein: 1992, 74)

Work can help contribute to a woman's sense of positive self-esteem as well as her perception of well-being. Nathanson (1980) reported that employment was positively related to self-esteem and the effect was most marked upon women who had few other avenues to enhance their self-esteem. Women with disabilities are likely to have lower levels of education and hence lower self-esteem; therefore, it is likely that this finding is especially applicable to them. Kutner and Gray's (1981) study of women with chronic renal failure found that women who were employed had lower depression scores than women who were homemakers. Furthermore, for many women work also provides a social network; therefore, disruption of employment also disrupts social interactions (Brintnell et al.: 1994).

Women with recently acquired disabilities should think carefully about the type of work they would like to do, being realistic about their physical abilities and their stamina. Vocational assessment and counseling may prove useful to women whose conditions require a position change. Physical location of the place of employment, transportation, and work schedule are all important considerations regarding a particular position.

The Americans with Disabilities Act requires that employers make "reasonable accommodations" for people with disabilities (see Chapter 3, "Laws that Affect Women with Disabilities"). Advances in technology, especially in computer technology that is the core of most office work, have produced a variety of adapted equipment that enables even those with the most limited mobility to continue working. Women with minimal mobility can control their environment through the use of switches, headpointers, joysticks, and sip-and-puff switches; these devices are used in conjunction with special software or adapted hardware. For example, women with high quadriplegia are able to turn electrical devices on and off through the use of a sip-and-puff device. Switches that may be operated by a toe, a foot, or a hand permit entry of data into computers. Headpointers are attached to a headset and consist of pointers with rubber tips that are used to control keys on the keyboard. Joysticks enable women with limited motion to simulate the movement of a mouse.

Speech recognition systems enable women who are severely limited in their mobility to use personal computers in a variety of situations. These systems recognize the user's voice as an alternative way of entering data into computers and may be used to write and to carry out conversations, both on the job and in other settings.

Barrier-free design ensures that women with disabilities can enter and exit the building easily and safely; that bathroom facilities, water fountains, and employee dining rooms are accessible; that aisles and entryways are wide enough to accommodate wheelchairs; that ramps are placed where needed; and that floor coverings are amenable to the use of wheelchairs. Special paint or grit strip paint applied to slippery surfaces or inclines reduces the risk of accidents. Mirrors mounted at hallway intersections and see-through panels in doors may help prevent accidents for employees traveling in wheelchairs. Elevator buttons, public telephones, and light switches should also be accessible to people who use wheelchairs. Staff members who are not disabled should be assigned the responsibility for helping women with disabilities to exit the building in case of an emergency, such as a fire, bomb threat, or toxic leak.

The space underneath the desk should be large enough to accommodate a wheelchair; file cabinets should be lateral so that they are within reach. Special desks and workstations are available to accommodate wheelchairs and adjust to the required height of the user. Where carpets are used, they should be low level pile to allow for easier mobility, and elevators should be large enough to accommodate wheelchairs. Some individuals use standing wheelchairs that offer flexibility in adapting to the workplace as well as improving circulation, reducing pressure sores, and allowing users to make direct eye contact with colleagues without looking up from a seated position.

Transportation has often been a barrier to employment for women with disabilities. Some women with disabilities may be able to operate their own automobiles or vans. Many car manufacturers offer specially adapted vans to carry wheelchairs. Some of these companies also have special purchase or loan programs for people with disabilities. General Motors, Ford, Saturn, and Chrysler offer financial assistance for the purchase of adaptive equipment such as hand controls, a ramp, or lifts to be installed in vehicles (see "ORGANIZATIONS" section under Recreation and Travel in this chapter). Public transportation systems may have regular buses with special equipment to lift wheelchairs, or they may offer transportation in vehicles specially designed for people with disabilities. The entry from the parking lot should provide enough space for wheelchairs to be removed from the vehicle. Level ground or ramps should lead into the building.

Women who require continued medical supervision to manage their conditions should be allowed time to schedule doctors' appointments. Flexibility is often the key, enabling women to work through lunch or later hours one day in order to take time off for medical care another day. Employers who cooperate to accommodate the special needs of women with disabilities and chronic conditions will contribute to a more productive workforce.

References

Brintnell, E. Sharon et al.
1994   "Disruption of Life Roles Following Injury: Impact on Women's Social Networks" Work 4:2:137-146
Hillyer, Barbara
1993   Feminism and Disability Norman, OK: University of Oklahoma Press
Kutner, Nancy G. and Heather L. Gray
1981   "Women and Chronic Renal Failure: Some Neglected Issues" Journal of Sociology and Social Welfare 8:2:320-332
McNeil, John M.
1993   Americans with Disabilities 1991-1992 Washington DC: U.S. Bureau of the Census Current Population Reports P70-33
Nathanson, Constance A.
1980   "Social Roles and Health Status among Women: The Significance of Employment" Social Science and Medicine 14A:463-471
Sherr Klein, Bonnie
1992   "We Are Who You Are" Ms. III(November/December):3:70-74
U.S. Department of Labor Women's Bureau
1992   "Women with Work Disabilities" Facts on Working Women March, No. 92.2

# ORGANIZATIONS

Association of Part-Time Professionals (APTP)
7700 Leesburg Pike, Suite 216
Falls Church, VA 22043
(703) 734-7975

A membership organization that works to promote part-time work and flexible work options. Among its goals are equitable compensation, benefits, and work schedules. Individual membership, $20.00, includes monthly newsletter "Working Options."

Equal Employment Opportunity Commission (EEOC)
1801 L Street, NW, 10th Floor
Washington, DC 20507
(800) 669-3362 to order publications
(800) 669-4000 to speak to an investigator
(800) 800-3302 (TT)
In Washington, DC, (202) 275-7377    (202) 275-7518 (TT)            BBS (202) 514-6193

Responsible for developing regulations and enforcing the employment section of the ADA. Copies of its regulations are available in standard print, large print, braille, computer disk, and on audiocassette. Provides guidance to federal agencies in their affirmative action programs for hiring and promoting people with disabilities and processes complaints filed by individuals.

Job Accommodation Network (JAN)
West Virginia University
918 Chestnut Ridge Road, Suite 1
PO Box 6080
Morgantown, WV 26506-6080
(800) 526-7234                      (800) 232-9675 (V/TT)
In Canada, (800) 526-2262          FAX (304) 293-5407            BBS: (800) 342-5526
e-mail: jan@jan.icdi.wvu.edu       http://www.jan.wvu.edu

Maintains database of products that facilitate accommodation in the workplace. Provides information to employers about practical accommodations which enable them to employ individuals with disabilities.

9to5, National Association of Working Women
238 West Wisconsin Ave, Suite 700
Milwaukee WI 53203
(800) 522-0925 jobs problem hot-line  (414) 274-0925            FAX (414) 272-2870

Works on policy issues that affect working women, such as pregnancy discrimination and sexual harassment. Provides legal advice and offers a hot-line to help women who have job related problems. Membership, $25.00, includes "9to5 Newsletter."

President's Committee on Employment of People with Disabilities (PCEPD)
1331 F Street, NW
Washington, DC 20004
(202) 376-6200                    (202) 376-6206 (TT)                    FAX (202) 376-6219

A federal agency that fosters communication among the various state and local agencies that work toward improved employment opportunities for people with disabilities, labor unions, and private enterprise. Holds an annual conference and sponsors studies.

Rehabilitation Engineering and Assistive Technology Society of North America/RESNA
1700 North Moore Street, Suite 1540
Arlington, VA 22209-1903
(703) 524-6686                    (703) 524-6639 (TT)                    FAX (703) 524-6630
http://www.resna.org/resna/reshome.htm

Multidisciplinary professional membership organization for people involved with improving technology for people with disabilities. Conducts a variety of projects, including research in the area of assistive technology and rehabilitation technology service delivery and technical assistance to statewide programs to develop technology. Membership, regular, $120.00; institutional, $275.00; corporate, $525.00; varying fees for students; includes semiannual journal, "Assistive Technology" and "RESNA News." Nonmember subscription to "Assistive Technology," individuals, $49.95; institutions, $62.00.

Rehabilitation Technology Associates
Barron Drive, Box 1004
Institute, WV 25112-1004
(304) 766-2680                    (304) 766-2697 (TT)                    FAX (304) 766-2689
e-mail: rta@rtc2.icdi.wvu.edu

A membership organization for professionals in the rehabilitation field who use technology in the performance of their jobs. Holds an annual meeting. Membership is free. Publishes quarterly newsletter, "On Line," available in standard print, on audiocassette, and on PC disk.

United Cerebral Palsy Association
Assistive Technology Funding and Systems Change Project
1660 L Street, NW
Washington, DC 20036
(800) 827-0093

Provides information about funding sources for assistive technology and refers individuals to local resources.

Vocational Rehabilitation Services
Veterans Benefits Administration
Department of Veterans Affairs (VA)
810 Vermont Avenue, NW
Washington, DC 20420
(202) 233-6496

Provides education, rehabilitation, and independent living services to veterans with service related disabilities through offices located in every state as well as regional centers, medical centers, and insurance centers. Medical services are provided at VA Medical Centers, Outpatient Clinics, Domiciliaries, and Nursing Homes.

Wider Opportunities for Women (WOW)
815 15th Street, NW, Suite 916
Washington, DC 20005
(202) 638-3143                      FAX (202) 638-3143

Works to achieve economic independence and equity for women and girls. Leads the Women's Workforce Network, a coalition of programs throughout the country that provide counseling, information, and training to women who are seeking jobs. Free publications list. Membership, $25.00, includes semi-annual newsletter "Women at Work."

Women's Bureau
U.S. Department of Labor
200 Constitution Avenue, NW
Washington, DC 20210
(800) 827-5335                (800) 326-2577 (TT)                (202) 219-6610
http://www.dol.gov/dol/wb/

Works to improve working conditions for women. Publishes brochures on subjects related to employment, such as "Disability Discrimination," "Family and Medical Leave," "Sexual Harassment," "Age Discrimination," "Pregnancy Discrimination," and "Wage Discrimination." All are free. The Fair Pay Clearinghouse, (800) 347-3741, offers publications and lists resources in U.S.

Adapting PCs for Disabilities
by Joseph J. Lazzaro
Addison-Wesley-Longman Publishing Company
1 Jacob Way
Reading, MA 01867
(800) 447-2226                              (617) 944-3700

This book describes how PCs can be adapted for use by individuals with physical, sensory, or cognitive impairments.  It discusses hardware, software, and Internet resources, lists equipment vendors, and provides information on the Technology Act and the Americans with Disabilities Act. Includes a CD-ROM edition of the text with adaptive software programs and a text file viewer. $39.95

Americans with Disabilities Act: Questions and Answers
Equal Employment Opportunity Commission  (EEOC)
1801 L Street, NW, 10th Floor
Washington, DC 20507
(800) 669-4000                         (800) 669-3362 publication orders
(202) 275-7377                         (202) 275-7518 (TT)
FAX (513) 791-2954                     BBS (202) 514-6193

This booklet's question and answer format provides explanations of the ADA, including  employment issues.  Large print, audiocassette, braille, and through a bulletin board service.  Free

Careers and the Disabled
Equal Opportunity Publications
1160 East Jericho Turnpike, Suite 200
Huntington, NY 11743
(516) 421-9421

This magazine features career guidance articles, role model profiles, and lists of companies looking for qualified job candidates.  Published three times per year; pre-paid subscription, $10.00; invoiced, $12.00.

Computer Resources for People with Disabilities
Alliance for Technology Access
2175 East Francisco Boulevard, Suite L
San Rafael, CA 94901
(800) 455-7970                    (415) 455-0491 (TT)          FAX (415) 455-0654
e-mail: atafta@aol.com           http://www.ataccess.org

This book describes assistive technology and discusses what to consider when making a purchase, the support team members that can provide assistance, and information on sources of funding for purchases.  Second edition.  Softcover, $17.95; spiral bound, $22.95; ASCII disk, $22.95.

Key Changes
Fanlight Productions
47 Halifax Street
Boston, MA 02130
(800) 937-4113                    (617) 542-0980                    FAX (617) 542-8838
e-mail: fanlight@tiac.net         http://www.fanlight.com

This videotape portrays Lisa Thorson, a vocalist who experienced a spinal cord injury and continues performing in her chosen profession. 28 minutes. Purchase, $195.00; rental, $50.00; plus $9.00 shipping and handling.

Meeting the Needs of Employees with Disabilities
Resources for Rehabilitation
33 Bedford Street, Suite 19A
Lexington, MA 02173
(617) 862-6455                    FAX (617) 861-7517

This book provides information to help people with disabilities retain or obtain employment. Information on government programs and laws, supported employment, training programs, environmental adaptations, and the transition from school to work are included. Chapters on mobility, vision, and hearing and speech impairments include information on organizations, products, and services that enable employers to accommodate the needs of employees with disabilities. $42.95 plus $5.00 shipping and handling. (See order form on last page of this book.)

Part of the Team - People with Disabilities in the Workforce
National Easter Seal Society
230 West Monroe Street, Suite 1800
Chicago, IL 60606
(800) 221-6827                    (312) 726-6200                    (312) 726-4258 (TT)
FAX (312) 726-1494               e-mail: nessinfo@seals.com        http://www.seals.com

This videotape profiles ten individuals who have overcome physical barriers to employment with cooperation and communication with their employers. $15.00 (1/2" format); $25.00 (3/4" format); also available with open captions at no additional cost.

The Workplace Workbook 2.0
by James Mueller
HRD Press
22 Amherst Road
Amherst, MA 01002
(800) 822-2801                    (413) 253-3488                    FAX (413) 253-3490

A guide to workplace accommodation and technology for employees with and without disabilities. Includes illustrations and resources. $49.95 plus $5.00 shipping and handling.

## VENDORS OF ASSISTIVE DEVICES

Listed below are manufacturers of assistive devices that can help women with disabilities in the workplace.

Don Johnston, Inc.
PO Box 639
1000 North Rand Road, Building 115
Wauconda, IL 60084-0639
(800) 999-4660    (847) 526-2682    FAX (847) 526-4177
http://www.donjohnston.com

Mail order catalogue of devices that enable individuals with disabilities to have alternative access to computer operations.  Produces Ke:nx, which provides a variety of alternative modes to access the Macintosh computer, using switches, specially designed keyboards, etc.

Dragon Systems
320 Nevada Street
Newton, MA 02160
(800) 825-5897    (617) 965-5200    FAX (617) 527-0372

Manufactures Dragon Dictate, a speech recognition system that enables individuals to speak instead of typing to dictate their work into a computer.  Requires a PC.

IBM Independence Series
Building #904-Internal ZIP 9448
11400 Burnet Road
Austin, TX 78758
(800) 426-4832    (800) 426-4833 (TT) for information
(800) 426-3388    (800) 426-3383 (TT) for orders
For calls from Canada, (800) 465-7999

The IBM Keyguard attaches to either the IBM Enhanced or Space Saving keyboard to expose and isolate individual keys for users with poor hand control.  IBM Screen Magnifier and Screen Reader software provides computer access to people with vision impairments.  The IBM VoiceType family of products allows users to dictate directly into computer programs such as Microsoft Word; call (800) 825-5263 for more information.

In Touch Systems
11 Westview Road
Spring Valley, NY 10977
(800) 332-6244    (914) 354-7431

Manufactures the Magic Wand Keyboard, a miniature keyboard for PC's or Apple computers for individuals with restricted hand movement.  Uses a hand-held wand or mouthstick to select keys.

LC Technologies
9455 Silver King Court
Fairfax, VA 22031
(800) 733-5284                   (703) 385-7133                   FAX (703) 385-7137
http://www.lctinc.com

Manufactures the Eyegaze Computer System which enables individuals with severe mobility impairments to use their eyes to control devices in their environment, to use the telephone, and to use a computer. A 25 minute videotape demonstration of the Eyegaze Computer System is available. Free

Madenta Communications
9411A 20th Avenue
Edmonton, Alberta T6N 1E5 Canada
(800) 661-8406                   (403) 450-8926                   FAX (403) 988-6182
e-mail: madenta@madenta.com     http://www.madenta.com

Produces adaptive software for Macintosh computers that provides keyboard, pointing, voice, and single switch access for individuals with mobility impairment. Also produces environmental controls to use with PC's and Macintosh.

Microsystems Software
600 Worcester Road
Framingham, MA 01702
(800) 828-2600                   (508) 879-9000                   FAX (508) 626-8515
http://www.microsys.com

Produces software that enables users with mobility impairments to access computers and use telephone systems. HandiWORD enables users with limited keyboard abilities to use popular word processing and spreadsheet programs available for DOS and Windows. HandiKEY software allows users to access DOS and Windows 3.1 with switching devices, such as a joystick, headmouse, or trackball; a deluxe version drives a speech synthesizer. HandiPHONE is a computer controlled telephone system that enables users to access telephones without the use of their hands. MAGic is screen magnification software for DOS and MAGic Deluxe is for Windows. Large print or audiocassette user guide available for MAGic Deluxe. Microsystems Software bulletin board, (508) 875-8009.

Prentke Romich
1022 Heyl Road
Wooster, OH 44691
(800) 262-1984                   (330) 262-1984                   FAX (330) 263-4829

Produces alternative computer access devices, including a variety of switches, special no-touch keyboards, and disk guides. Provides training in the use of their products.

Touch Turner
443 View Ridge Drive
Everett, WA 98203
(206) 252-1541                   FAX (206) 259-4390

Manufactures a product that turns pages of books or magazines, available with a variety of switches. Operates on batteries or with electrical adaptor.

Voice Connexion
17971 Skypark Circle, Suite F
Irvine, CA 92614
(714) 261-2366                    FAX (714) 261-8563
e-mail: voicecnx@aol.com          http://www.access1.com/vcx

Manufactures voice recognition and speech synthesis hardware and software for PC's and compatibles.

# HOUSING AND ENVIRONMENTAL ADAPTATIONS

Housing plays an important role in a woman's ability to remain independent. Most women with disabilities will opt to live in their own home whenever possible. Often this requires financial assistance, household help, environmental modifications, or moving to a more accessible building. The government has provided a number of programs to assist people with disabilities with affordable housing and to protect them from discrimination.

The *Fair Housing Act of 1988* prohibits discrimination in housing due to race, religion, gender, family status, disability, and national origin. It is enforced by the Department of Housing and Urban Development (HUD). It applies to sale and rental of most housing and mortgage lending. New buildings constructed after March 13, 1991 that have an elevator and four or more units must be accessible to individuals with disabilities. Tenants with disabilities have the legal right to make modifications to rental housing at their own expense in order to meet their needs. However, the residence must be restored to its original condition "within reason" when the tenant moves. In addition, HUD has established programs to house individuals with disabilities who are homeless. When individuals with disabilities file a complaint, HUD will provide interpreters, materials on cassette or in braille, and assistance in reading and filling out forms.

*Home Equity Conversion Mortgages*, sometimes called reverse mortgages, allow elders to convert the equity in their homes into cash that will enable them to meet housing expenses. These mortgages are insured by HUD in the event that the lender defaults. The reverse mortgage does not have to be repaid until the mortgagee moves or dies. Homeowners must be age 62 or older, occupy their own home as a principal residence, and own the home free and clear or nearly so. Reverse mortgage payment options include "tenure," monthly payments to homeowners as long as they use their homes as principal residences; "term," which provides monthly payments for a specified period; and "line-of-credit," which allows homeowners to draw on their equity up to a maximum amount. HUD USER [(800) 245-2691] can provide more information on this program.

*Public housing* is a major resource for women with disabilities and older women with low income. *Section 8* Certificates and Vouchers provide federal subsidies to income-eligible households to help defray housing costs in the private rental market. Section 8 subsidies may also be used in group residences. Local public housing authorities administer the program. *Section 803* of the National Affordable Housing Act of 1990, HOPE for Elderly Independence, combines tenant-based rental housing certificates and rental vouchers with supportive services to enable frail elders who have not been receiving any form of housing assistance to continue living in the community.

*Section 202* Supportive Housing for the Elderly funds consumer cooperatives and private nonprofit organizations to increase the supply of housing with supportive services for individuals with disabilities and elders. Those who qualify based on age must be age 62 or older and have very low incomes.

Women who feel that they have experienced discrimination in housing may file complaints with HUD or a state or local fair housing agency, or they may file a civil suit.

Other housing options for women with disabilities include assisted living facilities, such as board and care homes, adult care homes, and residential care facilities. Many cities have residential hotels for older women with services, such as housekeeping, security, and social activities. Continuing care retirement communities provide housing choices ranging from independent apartment living with services, such as congregate meals and activities, to 24-hour nursing care. Shared housing programs include shared group residences and programs which match elders who need some assistance to remain at home with younger people who need inexpensive housing. Accessory housing, independent housing units built on to single family homes or erected on the property of a single family home, is another option for elders who wish to live independently but need supportive services.

Women with disabilities who wish to remain in their own homes may find that environmental adaptations enable them to do so. For example, the installation of ramps, elevators, and special lifts to climb the stairs may be sufficient for those with mobility impairments. Lowered kitchen counters and appliances facilitate cooking for women who use wheelchairs. Other adaptive design features include accessible routes, light switches, electrical outlets, and thermostats; bathrooms with walls sturdy enough to install grab bars; and kitchens and bathrooms with sufficient space to maneuver wheelchairs.

Many architects now specialize in designing buildings and dwelling units that meet the needs of people with disabilities. The state office on disability, the architectural access board, or the local or state professional society of architects should be able to provide a list of qualified architects.

ABLEDATA
8455 Colesville Road, Suite 935
Silver Spring, MD 20910-3319
(800) 227-0216                    (301) 588-9284                    (301) 495-5626 (TT)
FAX (301) 587-1967               BBS (301) 589-3563
http://www.abledata.com

A database of disability-related products for personal care, recreation, and transportation. First 20 items from database searches, free; a fee is charged for longer searches. Also available on CD-ROM, $25.00; monthly update files, $25.00 per release cycle (four updates). Also available on the Internet at no charge.


Architectural and Transportation Barriers Compliance Board (ATBCB)
1331 F Street, NW, Suite 1000
Washington, DC 20004-1111
(800) 872-2253                    (800) 993-2822 (TT)               (202) 272-5434
(202) 272-5449 (TT)              FAX (202) 272-5447
http://www.access-board.gov     BBS (202) 272-5448

A federal agency charged with developing standards for accessibility. Provides technical assistance, sponsors research, and distributes publications. Publishes a free quarterly newsletter, "Access America," and a free bimonthly newsletter, "Access Currents." Publications available in standard print, large print, braille, audiocassette, and computer disk.


Association of Home Appliance Manufacturers
20 North Wacker Drive
Chicago, IL 60606
(312) 984-5800

Provides referral to the major home appliance manufacturers for information on modifications for their products. Distributes "Do Your PART (Protect Against Range Tipping), a booklet describing safety measures to avoid kitchen accidents. Free


Center for Universal Design
North Carolina State University
Box 8613
Raleigh, NC 27695-8613
(800) 647-6777                    (919) 515-3082 (V/TT)            FAX (919) 515-3023
e-mail: cahd@ncsu.edu

A federally funded research and training center that works toward improving housing for people with disabilities. Provides technical assistance, training, and publications. Has established Remodelers' Referral Network to help individuals find contractors who specialize in home modifications.

Fair Housing Information Clearinghouse
Department of Housing and Urban Development (HUD)
PO Box 9146
McLean, VA 22102
(800) 343-3442                    (800) 483-2209 (TT)                    FAX (703) 821-2098

Distributes information about federal laws and regulations and other educational materials in support of federal laws that prohibit discrimination in housing. Many brochures are free; newsletter subscription, free. Information kit and publications list, free. Individuals who feel that they have been discriminated against should call the National HUD Discrimination Hotline, (800) 669-9777; (800) 927-9275 (TT).

GE Answer Center
9500 Williamsburg Plaza
Louisville, KY 40222
(800) 626-2000                    (800) 833-4322 (TT)

This consumer information center provides assistance to individuals with disabilities as well as to the general public. Appliance controls marked with braille or raised dots are available for individuals who are blind or visually impaired, free. Two brochures, "Appliance Help for Those with Special Needs," and "Basic Kitchen Planning for the Physically Handicapped," are free. The center is open 24 hours per day, seven days a week.

National Association of Home Builders (NAHB)
National Research Center, Economics and Policy Analysis Division
400 Prince George's Boulevard
Upper Marlboro, MD 20772-8731
(301) 249-4000                    FAX (301) 249-0305

Produces publications and provides training on housing and special needs. "Directory of Accessible Building Products 1996" describes commercially available products of use to individuals with disabilities. $4.00

National Kitchen & Bath Association
687 Willow Grove Street
Hackettstown, NJ 07840
(908) 852-0033                    FAX (908) 852-1695

Produces technical manuals on universal design for kitchens and bathrooms, a sourcebook for products, and directories of certified designers and dealers.

Office for Elderly and Handicapped People
Department of Housing and Urban Development (HUD)
451 7th Street, SW
Washington, DC 20410
(202) 708-2730                    FAX (202) 708-1300

Operates programs to make housing accessible, including loans for developers of independent living and group homes and loan and mortgage insurance for rehabilitation of single or multifamily units. Publishes "A Guide to Publications and Services," free; "Adaptable Housing," which offers general and technical information on accessible housing, $4.00; "Fair Housing Amendments Act of 1988: A Selected Resource Guide," $4.00; "Options for Elderly Homeowners: A Guide to Reverse Mortgages and Their Alternatives," $10.00; and a newsletter, "Recent Research Results," free. HUD publications are available from HUD USER, PO Box 6091, Rockville, MD 20849; (800) 245-2691; in MD, (301) 251-5154.

Office of Fair Housing and Equal Opportunity
Department of Housing and Urban Development (HUD)
451 7th Street, SW
Washington, DC 20410
(800) 669-9777                          (800) 927-9275 (TT)

Enforces the Fair Housing Act and distributes publications that explain the Act and how to file a housing discrimination complaint.

# PUBLICATIONS AND TAPES

Adapting the Home for the Physically Challenged
A/V Health Services
PO Box 61031
Raleigh, NC 27661
(540) 389-4339                     FAX (919) 872-6888

This videotape helps individuals who use wheelchairs or walkers to modify their homes. Ramp construction and modifications for every room are explained. 30 minutes. $89.95 plus $2.00 shipping and handling.

Building a Ramp
by John W. Henson
Independent Living Resource Center, Inc.
PO Box 55127
Little Rock, AR 72225

This manual provides practical guidelines for ramp construction, including choice of site, materials, and step-by-step instructions. Large print. $10.00

A Consumer's Guide to Home Adaptation
The Adaptive Environments Center
374 Congress Street, Suite 301
Boston, MA 02210
(617) 695-1225 (V/TT)               FAX (617) 482-8099

A workbook that enables people with disabilities to plan the modifications necessary to adapt their homes. Describes how to widen doorways, lower countertops, etc. $12.00

Designs for Independent Living and Tools for Independent Living
Appliance Information Service (AIS)
Whirlpool Corporation
Administrative Center
Benton Harbor, MI 49022
(800) 253-1301

These brochures provide information on adaptations for the home environment and major appliances. Free

The Do-Able Renewable Home
by John P. S. Salmen
American Association of Retired Persons (AARP)
Consumer Affairs-Program Department
601 E Street, NW
Washington, DC 20049
(800) 424-3410               (202) 434-2277               http://www.aarp.org

This book describes how elders with disabilities can modify their homes for independent living. Room-by-room modifications are accompanied by illustrations.  Free

Eighty-eight Easy-To-Make Aids for Older People & for Special Needs
by Don Caston
Hartley & Marks Publishers
Box 147
Point Roberts, WA 98281
(206) 945-2017                          FAX (604) 738-1913

This book provides practical adaptations for the home with step-by-step instructions.  U.S., $12.95 plus $3.00 shipping and handling; Canada, $14.95 plus $3.00 shipping and handling.

Fair Housing Accessibility Guidelines
Fair Housing Information Clearinghouse
PO Box 9146
McLean, VA 22102
(800) 343-3442                          (800) 290-1617 (TT)

This videotape shows how the Fair Housing Act and Accessibility Guidelines affect housing construction and depicts design techniques and construction methods that may be used in new construction.  $15.00

Fair Housing: It's Your Right
Office of Fair Housing and Equal Opportunity
Department of Housing and Urban Development
Room 5240
Washington, DC 20410
(800) 669-9777                          (800) 927-9275 (TT)

This booklet explains the provisions of the Fair Housing Act, including how to file a complaint, what to expect in a complaint investigation, and how to file suit if necessary.  Includes housing discrimination complaint form.  Free

Guide to Independent Living for People with Arthritis
Arthritis Foundation
1314 Spring Street, NW
Atlanta, GA 30309
(800) 283-7800                  (404) 872-7100                  FAX (404) 872-0457
http://www@arthritis.org

Although written for individuals with arthritis, this book contains photographs of hundreds of adaptive aids that enable individuals with other disabilities to live independently.  Product descriptions, hints for use, and names and addresses of manufacturers are provided.  $10.00

Homemade Money: Consumers' Guide to Home Equity Conversion
American Association of Retired Persons (AARP)
Consumer Affairs-Program Department
601 E Street, NW
Washington, DC 20049
(800) 424-3410                    (202) 434-2277                    http://www.aarp.org

This publication provides information on a program that allows older individuals to convert home equity into funds used to meet their housing expenses.  Free

Home Safety Checklist for Older Consumers
U.S. Consumer Product Safety Commission
Washington, DC  20207
(800) 638-2772

This booklet provides information on simple, inexpensive repairs and safety recommendations.  Also available in Spanish.  Free

Homes for Everyone, Universal Design Principles in Practice
HUD USER
PO Box 6091
Rockville, MD 20849
(800) 245-2691                    (800) 483-2209 (TT)                FAX (301) 251-5767
e-mail: huduser@aspensys.com      http://www.huduser.org

This book shows how universal design was used in building or remodeling 16 single-family homes.  Includes photographs, drawings, and floor plans.  $15.00

Housing and Support Services for Physically Disabled Persons in Canada
Canadian Rehabilitation Council for the Disabled (CRCD)
45 Sheppard Avenue East, Suite 801
Toronto, Ontario M2N 5W9  Canada
(416) 250-7490 (V/TT)             FAX (416) 229-1371

This book lists accessible housing options and other support services for people who live in Canada.  Also available in French.  Members, $20.00; nonmembers, $26.00; plus $3.00 shipping and handling, Canadian funds.

The Less Challenging Home
Appliance Information Service
Whirlpool Corporation
Benton Harbor, MI 49022
(800) 253-1301                    (800) 334-6889 (TT)

This booklet provides suggestions for incorporating accessible design when building or remodeling kitchens and bathrooms.  Describes building materials and appliances and includes charts indicating appliance features that are helpful to users with disabilities.  Free

Residential Remodeling and Universal Design: Making Homes More Comfortable and Accessible
HUD USER
PO Box 6091
Rockville, MD 20849
(800) 245-2691 (800) 483-2209 (TT) FAX (301) 251-5767
e-mail: huduser@aspensys.com http://www.huduser.org

This resource guide provides technical assistance to homeowners for design and installation of accessible fixtures, appliances, lighting, and other modifications. $5.00

Selecting Retirement Housing
American Association of Retired Persons (AARP)
601 E Street, NW
Washington, DC 20049
(800) 424-3410 (202) 434-2277 http://www.aarp.org

This publication describes retirement housing options and what to look for in housing contracts. It provides worksheets to help elders determine what option meets their needs and financial situation. Free

Shared Housing for the Elderly
by Dale Jaffe (ed.)
Greenwood Publishing Group
88 Post Road West
Westport, CT 06881
(800) 225-5800 (203) 226-3571 FAX (203) 222-1502
e-mail: prices@info.greenwood.com http://www.greenwood.com

A collection of articles about the advantages and problems of shared housing programs. $55.00 plus $3.00 shipping and handling.

Universal Design: Housing for the Lifespan of All People
Department of Housing and Urban Development (HUD)
Office of Public Affairs
Washington, DC 20410-0050

This book describes no-cost and low-cost options for accessible housing. $5.00

What Does Fair Housing Mean to People with Disabilities?
Office of Fair Housing and Equal Opportunity
Department of Housing and Urban Development
451 7th Street, SW
Washington, DC 20410
(800) 669-9777 (800) 927-9275 (TT)

This booklet describes the Fair Housing Act and the rights of individuals with disabilities, including definitions and examples of "reasonable accommodation" and building modifications, where to get help and how to file a complaint. $2.50

<u>Your Home, Your Choice: A Workbook for Older People and Their Families</u>
American Association of Retired Persons (AARP)
601 E Street, NW
Washington, DC 20049
(800) 424-3410                    (202) 434-2277                    http://www.aarp.org

This booklet provides checklists for assessing the home and describes supportive housing alternatives such as housesharing, congregate housing, and retirement homes.  Free

# VENDORS OF ASSISTIVE DEVICES

Listed below are manufacturers of assistive devices and mail order catalogues that specialize in devices for people with disabilities. Unless otherwise noted, catalogues include a variety of products and are free.

adaptAbility
Norwich Avenue
Box 515
Colchester, CT 06415-0515
(800) 266-8856                    FAX (800) 566-6678
e-mail: service@snswwide.com      http://www.snswwide.com

Aids that make dressing, eating, and bathing easier. Exercise and fitness activities and hot and cold therapy.

Arthritis Self Help Products
Aids for Arthritis, Inc.
3 Little Knoll Court
Medford, NJ 08055
(609) 654-6918

A mail order catalogue of products with dressing, bathing, and grooming aids and kitchen, housekeeping, and recreation equipment. Many of these products are useful for individuals with mobility impairments caused by other conditions.

Enrichments
PO Box 579
Hinsdale, IL 60521
(800) 323-5547                    FAX (800) 547-4333
http://www.sammonspreston.com

Independent Living Aids (ILA)
27 East Mall
Plainview, NY 11803
(800) 537-2118                    (516) 752-8080

Medela Inc.
PO Box 660
McHenry, IL 60051-0660
(800) 435-8316          (800) 995-7867          (815) 363-1166

Sells breastfeeding products, including electric breastpumps and the PedalPump, a manual breastpump accessory powered by foot pedal.

North Coast Medical Consumer Products Division
PO Box 6070
San Jose, CA 95150-6070
(800) 821-9319                          (800) 235-7054 (orders only)


The Right Start
5334 Sterling Center Drive
Westlake Village, CA 91361-4627
(800) 548-8531                          FAX (800) 762-5501


Sells products for infants and toddlers, nursing pillows that support the baby while breastfeeding, electric breastpumps, and hands-free baby carriers.


Sears Home HealthCare Catalog
Sears, Roebuck and Co.
20 Presidential Drive
Roselle, IL 60172
(800) 326-1750                          (800) 733-7249 (TT)


Sells practical and inexpensive devices, such as door knob covers, expanded hinges, reaching tools, and portable ramps. Sears Home HealthCare will file for Medicare reimbursement for customers. In-home or on-site service available.

# RECREATION AND TRAVEL

Both recreation and travel provide relief from tension, relaxation, and increased social interactions. Individuals who participate in recreational activities have an increased sense of self-worth and well-being. For individuals who are seriously ill, recreation diverts attention from the illness and provides opportunities for socialization. Some individuals with disabilities need assistance in order to continue with their favorite recreational pastimes. Others may develop an interest in new activities more appropriate to their current condition.

The Americans with Disabilities Act (ADA) of 1990 mandates accessibility to recreation facilities and athletic programs, from aerobic training classes and local parks to football stadiums and other venues. Advances in technology have led to the development of racing wheelchairs, special hand and foot prostheses, and adapted ski equipment such as sit-skis. The ADA also requires that fixed route buses and rail transportation be accessible and usable by individuals with disabilities. However, deadlines for implementation of the ADA's regulations vary from six to seven years for private intercity transit to as long as 20 years for Amtrak and commuter rail stations.

The Federal Aviation Administration requires each airline to submit a company wide policy for travelers with disabilities. Passengers may call ahead to request early boarding, special seating, or meals which meet dietary restrictions. Airport facilities are designed to offer accessible restrooms, elevators, electric carts or wheelchairs, and first aid stations. The Air Carrier Access Act of 1986 (ACAA) contains regulations that cover the needs of travelers with disabilities, such as access to commuter planes, accessible lavatories, wheelchair storage, and sensitivity training for all airline personnel. Contact the airlines to obtain a written statement of the special services they provide. Individuals who believe that their rights have been denied may file a complaint within 45 days of the incident with the Department of Transportation, Office of Consumer Affairs, 440 7th Street, SW, Room 10405, Washington, DC 20590, (202) 366-2220; (202) 765-7687 (TT).

Amtrak offers a 25% discount on a regular one-way coach fare for adults with disabilities. Passengers must present proof of disability, such as a certificate of legal blindness or a letter from a physician specifying the nature of the disability. Greyhound allows a passenger with a disability and a companion who will provide assistance in boarding/exiting the bus to travel for the price of a single adult fare. There is no charge for service dogs for individuals who are visually impaired, blind, or deaf.

Travel agencies that plan special trips for people with disabilities are available throughout the country. Many major hotel chains, airlines, and car rental companies provide special assistance to people with disabilities and often have special toll-free numbers for users of text telephones (TT's; formerly called telecommunication devices for the deaf or TDD's). Some companies offer specially trained travel companions to people with disabilities who need an escort. In the United States and Canada, many state and provincial tourism offices will provide information about accessible attractions for prospective visitors with disabilities. Auto clubs both here and abroad are also good sources for such information.

Individuals with disabilities and elders are eligible for special entrance passes to federal recreation facilities. The *Golden Access Passport* is a free lifetime pass available to any U.S. citizen or permanent resident, regardless of age, who is blind or permanently disabled. It admits the permit holder and passengers in a single, private, noncommercial vehicle to any parks, monuments, historic sites, recreation areas, and wildlife refuges which usually charge entrance fees. If the permit holder does not enter by car, the Passport admits the permit holder, spouse, and children. The permit holder is also entitled to a 50% discount on charges, such as camping, boat launching, and parking fees. Fees charged by private concessionaires are not discounted. Golden Access Passports are available only in person, with proof of disability, such as a certificate of legal blindness. Since the Passport is available at most federal recreation areas, it is not necessary to obtain one ahead of time. A *Golden Age Passport* offers the same benefits to persons aged 62 or older, with proof of age.

Rehabilitation hospitals and centers offer driver evaluation services such as clinical testing and observation to determine an individual's need for adaptive equipment or training. Many Department of Veterans Affairs Medical Centers (VAMC) offer driver evaluation services, driver training, and information services to veterans with disabilities through the Rehabilitation Medicine Service at their facilities. The Internal Revenue Service allows individuals to include in medical expenses the cost of special hand controls and other special equipment installed in a car to be used by a person with a disability. Individuals may also consider as a medical expense the difference between the cost of a car designed to hold a wheelchair and the cost of the car without modification. Contact the Internal Revenue Service (see "ORGANIZATIONS" section below) to obtain Publication 502 "Medical and Dental Expenses." Major automobile manufacturers offer reimbursement for adaptive equipment installed on new vehicles. Programs for special adaptive equipment offered by automobile manufacturers are listed in the "ORGANIZATIONS" section below.

# *ORGANIZATIONS*

Architectural and Transportation Barriers Compliance Board (ATBCB)
1331 F Street, NW, Suite 1000
Washington, DC 20004-1111

| | | |
|---|---|---|
| (800) 872-2253 | (800) 993-2822 (TT) | (202) 272-5434 |
| (202) 272-5449 (TT) | FAX (202) 272-5447 | |
| http://www.access-board.gov | BBS (202) 272-5448 | |

Maintains a database on accessible transportation, including a computerized, annotated bibliography. Publishes brochures on subjects such as "Air Carrier Policies on Transport of Battery Powered Wheelchairs." Computer bulletin board service is accessible 24 hours a day, (202) 272-5448.

Association of Driver Educators for the Disabled
PO Box 49
Edgerton, WI 53534
(608) 884-8833

Certifies members to conduct driver evaluation and training for individuals with disabilities.

Automobility
Chrysler Corporation
PO Box 3124
Bloomfield Hills, MI 48302

| | | |
|---|---|---|
| (800) 255-9877 | In Canada, (800) 265-6908 | FAX (810) 433-6343 |

Provides up to $1000 reimbursement (on eligible models) on the purchase of adaptive equipment for vehicles purchased to transport individuals who use wheelchairs and the purchase of alerting devices for people who are deaf or hard of hearing.

Disabled Sports USA (DS/USA)
451 Hungerford Drive, Suite 100
Rockville, Md 20850

| | | |
|---|---|---|
| (301) 217-0960 | (301) 217-0963 (TT) | FAX (301) 217-0968 |
| e-mail: dsusa@dsusa.org | http://www.dsusa.org/ ~ dsusa/dsusa.html | |

Nationwide network of chapters sponsors recreational activities such as skiing, camping, hiking, biking, horseback riding, and mountain climbing. Offers adaptive fitness instructor training to therapists, exercise instructors, and program directors. Membership, $25.00, includes subscription to newsletter, "Handicapped Sport Report."

Ford Mobility Motoring Program
PO Box 529
Bloomfield Hills, MI 48303

| | | |
|---|---|---|
| (800) 952-2248 | (800) 833-0312 (TT) | FAX (810) 333-2191 |
| In Canada, (800) 585-6985 | | |

This program funds adaptive equipment conversion up to $1000. Provides toll-free information line, list of assessment centers that determine equipment needs, and referrals to sources for additional assistance.

General Motors Mobility Assistance Center
PO Box 9011
Detroit, MI 48202
(800) 323-9935                    (800) 833-9935 (TT)              FAX (313) 974-4383
In Canada, (800) 263-3777 (English)   (800) 263-3830 (TT)

This program reimburses customers up to $1000 for vehicle modifications or adaptive driving devices for new or demo vehicles. Includes alerting devices for drivers who are deaf or hard of hearing such as emergency vehicle siren detectors and enhanced turn signal reminders.

Handicapped Scuba Association
1104 El Prado
San Clemente, CA 92672-4637
(714) 498-6128                    FAX (714) 498-6128

This organization trains and certifies scuba diving instructors to work with individuals with disabilities; teaches able-bodied divers to accompany divers with disabilities; and certifies divers with disabilities in "open water" diving. All contributors become members.

Internal Revenue Service (IRS)
(800) 829-1040                    (800) 829-4059 (TT)
telnet fedworld.gov               http://www.irs.ustreas.gov

The IRS provides technical assistance about tax credits and deductions related to accommodations for disabilities. To request Publication 502, "Medical and Dental Expenses," call (800) 829-3676; (800) 829-4059 (TT).

Mobility International USA (MIUSA)
PO Box 10767
Eugene, OR 97440
(541) 343-1284 (V/TT)             FAX (541) 343-6812              e-mail: miusa@igc.apc.org

Promotes the participation of youth and young adults with disabilities in international and educational exchange programs, such as workcamps, conferences, and internships. Annual membership, $25.00, includes quarterly newsletter, "Over the Rainbow." Newsletter only, $15.00.

National Foundation of Wheelchair Tennis
940 Calle Amanecer, Suite B
San Clemente, CA 92673
(714) 361-3663                    FAX (714) 361-6603             http://www.nfwt.org

Provides tournaments for athletes with disabilities. Publishes monthly newsletter.

National Mobility Equipment Dealers Association
909 East Skagway Avenue
Tampa, FL 33604
(800) 833-0427                    (813) 932-8566                    FAX (813) 931-4683

The members of this organization are car dealers, manufacturers, driver evaluators, and insurance companies.  Provides local referrals to members who are adaptive equipment dealers and rates members' competencies in equipment installation and conversion.

National Park Service
Department of the Interior, Office of Public Affairs
PO Box 37127
Washington, DC 20013-7127

Operates the Golden Access Passport program for people who have disabilities.  Free brochure.

National Transportation Agency of Canada
Accessible Transportation Directorate
Ottawa, Ontario  K1A 0N9 Canada
In Canada, (800)  883-1813          (800) 669-5575 (TT)          (819) 997-6828
(819) 953-9705 (TT)                 FAX (819) 953-6019

A federal agency that enforces the National Transportation Act of 1987 and regulations aimed at removing barriers to travel for persons with disabilities.  Provides consultation, monitors compliance, and provides conflict resolution.  Provides publications for consumers in large print, audiocassette, braille, and on computer disk.  Free

North American Riding for the Handicapped Association (NARHA)
PO Box 33150
Denver, CO 80233
(800) 369-7433                    (303) 452-1212                    FAX (303) 252-4610

This professional association promotes therapeutic horseback riding for individuals with disabilities and accredits riding programs.  Membership, $35.00, includes membership directory and subscription to two newsletters, "NARHA Strides," published quarterly, and "NARHA News," published eight times a year.

Saturn Mobility Program
PO Box 3900
Peoria, IL 61612
(800) 522-5000                    (800) 833-6000 (TT)          http://www.saturn.com

This program reimburses customers up to $1000 for adaptive equipment costs when an eligible new Saturn is purchased or leased.

Society for the Advancement of Travel for the Handicapped (SATH)
347 Fifth Avenue, Suite 610
New York, NY 10016
(212) 447-0027                          FAX (212) 725-8253

Advocates for accessibility for individuals with disabilities and serves as a clearinghouse for information on barrier-free travel. Membership, individuals, $45.00; seniors and students, $25.00; includes quarterly newsletter, "Open World for Accessible Travel."

Wheelchair Sports, USA
3595 East Fountain Boulevard, Suite L-1
Colorado Springs, CO 80910
(719) 574-1150                          FAX (719) 574-9840

This organization provides opportunities for individuals who use wheelchairs to compete in team and individual sports at local, regional, national, and international levels. The sports are archery, track and field, basketball, fencing, quad rugby, racquetball, shooting, sled hockey, swimming, table tennis, waterskiing, and weightlifting. Membership, $25.00; includes semiannual newsletter.

Wheelers Accessible Van Rental
(800) 456-1371

Rents mini-vans accessible to wheelchair users throughout the country.

Wilderness Inquiry
1313 5th Street, SE, Box 84
Minneapolis, MN 55414-1546
(800) 728-0719 (V/TT)        In Minneapolis and St. Paul, (612) 379-3858 (V/TT)
FAX (612) 379-5972

Sponsors trips into wilderness areas for individuals with disabilities or chronic conditions. Request schedule of current trips.

# *PUBLICATIONS*

Accessible Gardening for People with Physical Disabilities
by Janeen R. Adil
Woodbine House
6510 Bells Mill Road
Bethesda, MD 20817
(800) 843-7323    (301) 897-3570    FAX (301) 897-5838
e-mail: woodbine85@aol.com

Written for people with a variety of mobility impairments, this book provides information on making existing gardens more accessible and creating new gardens. Sources for obtaining supplies are included. $16.95 plus $4.00 shipping and handling.

Access Travel: Airports
Consumer Information Center
PO Box 100
Pueblo, CO 81002
(719) 948-3334    BBS (202) 208-7679
e-mail: cic.info@pueblo.gsa.gov   http://www.gsa.gov/staff/pa/cic/cic.htm

This brochure lists facilities and services for people with disabilities in airport terminals worldwide. Free

Air Transportation Regulations
Accessible Transportation Directorate
National Transportation Agency of Canada
Ottawa, Ontario K1A 0N9 Canada
In Canada, (800) 883-1813  (800) 669-5575 (TT)  (613) 997-6828
(819) 953-9705 (TT)   FAX (819) 953-6019

This publication describes the services that travelers with disabilities must receive when traveling on large aircraft. Free. The Accessible Transportation Directorate also provides information on other types of accessible travel.

Directory of Travel Agencies for the Disabled $19.95
Travel for the Disabled: A Handbook of Travel Resources and 500 Worldwide Access Guides $19.95
by Helen Hecker
Twin Peaks Press
PO Box 129
Vancouver, WA 98666-0129
(800) 637-2256    (360) 694-2462    FAX (360) 696-3210

The "Directory" lists travel agents who specialize in arrangements for people with disabilities in the U.S., Canada, and abroad. The "Handbook" lists access guides and accessible places plus travel tips. Both titles available in standard print or on audiocassette. Shipping, $3.00 first book, $1.50 additional book.

Disability and Sport
by Karen P. DePauw and Susan J. Gavron
Human Kinetics
PO Box 5076
Champaign, IL 61825-5076
(800) 747-4457

This book reviews the development of the sports movement for individuals with disabilities. Describes sports modifications, lists disability sports organizations, discusses coaching athletes with disabilities, and provides information about publications. Includes biographies of athletes with disabilities. $35.00 plus $3.75 shipping and handling.

The Disabled Driver's Mobility Guide
Traffic Safety and Engineering
American Automobile Association (AAA)
1000 AAA Drive
Heathrow, FL 32746-5063
(407) 444-7962

This book provides information about adaptive equipment, driver training, and travel information services. $7.95

Easy Access to National Parks: The Sierra Club Guide for People with Disabilities
by Wendy Roth and Michael Tompane
Sierra Club Books
85 Second Street, 2nd Floor
San Francisco, CA 94105
(800) 935-1056                    (415) 977-5600                    FAX (415) 977-5793
http://www.sierraclub.org/books

This book reviews accessibility of 50 national parks for individuals with vision, hearing, or mobility impairments. $16.00 plus $4.00 shipping and handling. Available in braille on loan from the National Library Service for the Blind and Physically Handicapped (See page 29).

Fodor's Great American Vacations for Travelers with Disabilities
Random House
400 Hahn Road, PO Box 100
Westminster, MD 21157
(800) 293-2665                    (410) 848-1900                    FAX (410) 386-7013
http://www.randomhouse.com

This book describes accessibility features for individuals with mobility, hearing, and vision impairments available in 38 popular vacation destinations in the U.S. Includes hotels, restaurants, and attractions. U.S., $19.50; Canada, $27.00.

Handi-Travel: A Resource Book for Disabled and Elderly Travellers
by Cinnie Noble
Canadian Rehabilitation Council for the Disabled (CRCD)
45 Sheppard Avenue East, Suite 801
Toronto, Ontario M2N 5W9 Canada
(416) 250-7490 (V/TT)          FAX (416) 229-1371

Provides travel information about air, rail, bus, and ship transportation. Available in English and French. Members, $10.00; nonmembers, $12.95; plus $3.00 shipping and handling, Canadian funds for orders from Canada; U.S. funds for orders from outside Canada.

New Horizons for the Air Traveler with a Disability
Consumer Information Center
PO Box 100
Pueblo, CO 81002
(719) 948-3334                    BBS (202) 208-7679
e-mail: cic.info@pueblo.gsa.gov   http://www.gsa.gov/staff/pa/cic/cic.htm

This booklet describes accessibility requirements for accommodations, facilities, and services. Free

Sports 'N Spokes
2111 East Highland Avenue, Suite 180
Phoenix, AZ 85016-9611
(602) 224-0500

A bimonthly magazine that features articles about sports activities for people who use wheelchairs. U.S., $18.00; foreign, $21.00.

Travel Tips for People with Arthritis
Arthritis Foundation
PO Box 19000
Atlanta, GA 30326
(800) 283-7800                (404) 872-7100          FAX (404) 872-0457
http://www@arthritis.org

This booklet has advice for individuals who have difficulty walking or who use a cane or wheelchair. Suggestions on selection of accessible hotels, travel agents, and accessible transportation. Free

A World of Options for the 1990's: A Guide to International Educational Exchange, Community Service, and Travel for Persons with Disabilities
by Cindy Lewis and Susan Sygall
Mobility International USA (MIUSA)
PO Box 10767
Eugene, OR 97440
(541) 343-1284 (V/TT)          FAX (541) 343-6812          e-mail: miusa@igc.apc.org

Lists educational exchange programs, international workcamps, and accessible travel opportunities. Personal experiences are used to describe these programs. Members, $14.00; nonmembers, $16.00.

# VENDORS OF ASSISTIVE DEVICES

The following vendors sell assistive devices that help people with disabilities enjoy sports and recreational activities, such as swimming aids, fishing equipment, fitness equipment and home gyms, golf clubs, wheelchair ramps, bowling aids, and adapted games. Unless otherwise noted, the catalogues are free.

Abilitations
One Sportime Way
Atlanta, GA 30340
(800) 850-8602                    FAX (800) 850-8603

Access to Recreation, Inc.
PO Box 5072-430
Thousand Oaks, CA 91359-5072
(800) 634-4351                    FAX (805) 498-8186

adaptAbility
Norwich Avenue
Colchester, CT 06415-0515
(800) 243-9232                    FAX (800) 566-6678

Worldwide Games
PO Box 517
Colchester, CT 06415-0517
(800) 243-9232                    FAX (800) 566-6678

# Chapter 3

# LAWS THAT AFFECT WOMEN WITH DISABILITIES

*(For laws related to housing, see Chapter 2, "Coping with Daily Activities")*

Laws that affect women with disabilities cover a wide range of issues, including health care, financial benefits, rehabilitation, civil rights, transportation, access to public buildings, and employment. For those who are not specialists in the law, it is sometimes difficult to keep abreast of the laws and their amendments. At the same time, women with disabilities may be able to continue living independently if they are aware of their rights and know how to locate services and equipment provided by government programs or financial assistance to reimburse private providers.

In 1990, the *Americans with Disabilities Act* (ADA) was passed. Considered the most important piece of civil rights legislation in recent years, the ADA (P.L. 101-336) increases the steps employers must take to accommodate employees with disabilities and requires that new buses and rail vehicles, facilities, and public accommodations be accessible. The ADA defines disability as "a physical or mental impairment that substantially limits one or more of the major life activities..." [such as speaking, hearing, seeing, or walking]; "a record of such impairment;" or "being regarded as having such an impairment." Thus, individuals who have been cured of cancer or mental illness may still be regarded by others as having a disability and may experience discrimination. Others may have a physical condition that does not limit activity, such as disfiguring scars from injuries incurred in an automobile accident, but are regarded as disabled. Individuals in these situations are covered by the law.

The major provisions of the ADA are as follows:

 • Prohibits discrimination against individuals with disabilities who are otherwise qualified for employment and requires that employers make "reasonable accommodations." "Reasonable accommodations" include making existing facilities accessible and job restructuring (e.g., reassignment to a vacant position, modification of equipment, training, provision of interpreters and readers). Employers are protected from "undue hardship" in complying with this provision; the financial situation of the employer and the size and type of business are considered when determining whether an accommodation would constitute "undue hardship." This section was effective July 26, 1992 for employers with 25 or more employees and July 26, 1994 for employers with 15 or more employees. (For a more detailed discussion of the employment aspects of the ADA, see Meeting the Needs of Employees with Disabilities, described in "PUBLICATIONS AND TAPES" section below)

 • Prohibits discrimination by public entities (i.e., local and state governments) and requires that individuals with disabilities be entitled to the same rights and benefits of public programs as other individuals. This section was effective January 26, 1992.

 • Requires that bus and railroad transportation systems address the needs of individuals with disabilities by purchasing adapted equipment, modifying facilities, and providing special transportation services that are comparable to regular transportation services. Effective dates vary with the type of transportation system.

• Requires that public accommodations, businesses, and services be accessible to individuals with disabilities. Public accommodations are broadly defined to include places such as hotels and motels, theatres, museums, schools, shopping centers and stores, banks, restaurants, and professional service providers' offices. After January 26, 1993, most new construction for public accommodations must be accessible to individuals with disabilities.

• Mandates that telephone companies provide relay services 24 hours a day, seven days a week, for individuals with hearing or speech impairments. Relay services enable individuals who have text telephones (TT's; formerly called telecommunication devices for the deaf or TDD's) or another computer device that is capable of communicating across telephone lines to communicate with individuals who do not have such devices. This section was effective July 26, 1993.

Copies of the ADA and all federal laws are available from Senators and Representatives. Agencies charged with formulating regulations and standards include the Architectural and Transportation Barriers Compliance Board, the Department of Transportation, the Equal Employment Opportunity Commission, the Federal Communications Commission, and the Attorney General. Regulations for enforcing individual sections of the ADA are available from the federal agencies charged with promulgating them and in the "Federal Register" (see "PUBLICATIONS" section below). In addition, many private agencies that work with individuals with disabilities have copies of the ADA available for distribution to the public.

Other major laws that affect women with disabilities include the *Rehabilitation Act of 1973* (P.L. 93-112) and its amendments, which are the centerpieces of federal law related to rehabilitation. States must submit a vocational rehabilitation plan to the Rehabilitation Services Administration indicating how the designated state agency will provide vocational training, counseling, and diagnostic and evaluation services required by the law. Subsequent reauthorizations of and amendments to the Rehabilitation Act expanded the services provided under this law. For example, the "Client Assistance Program" authorizes states to inform clients and other persons with disabilities about all available benefits under the Act and to assist them in obtaining all remedies due under the law (P.L. 98-221). "Comprehensive Services for Independent Living" (P.L. 95-602) expands rehabilitation services to individuals with severe disabilities, regardless of their vocational potential, making services available to many people who are no longer in the work force. The Act broadly defines services as any "service that will enhance the ability of a handicapped individual to live independently or function within his family and community..." These services may include counseling, job placement, housing, funds to make the home accessible, funds for prosthetic devices, attendant care, and recreational activities.

*Section 503 of the Rehabilitation Act* requires any contractor that receives more than $2,500 in contracts from the federal government to take affirmative action to employ individuals with disabilities. The Office of Federal Contract Compliance Programs within the Department of Labor is responsible for enforcing this provision (see "ORGANIZATIONS" section below). *Section 504* prohibits any program that receives federal financial assistance from discriminating against individuals with disabilities who are otherwise eligible to benefit from their programs. Virtually all educational institutions are affected by this law, including private postsecondary institutions which receive federal financial assistance under a wide variety of programs. Programs must be physically accessible to individuals with disabilities, and construction begun after implementation of the regulations (June 3, 1977) must be designed so that it is in compliance with standard specifications for accessibility. Federal agencies must develop an affirmative action plan for hiring, placing, and promoting individuals with disabilities and for making their facilities accessible. The Civil Rights Division of the Department of Justice is responsible for enforcing this section.

The *Rehabilitation Act Amendments of 1992* (P.L. 102-569) establish state rehabilitation advisory councils composed of representatives of independent living councils, parents of children with disabilities, vocational rehabilitation professionals, and business; the role of these councils is to advise state vocational rehabilitation agencies and to prepare an annual report for the governor. The Amendments require that each state agency establish performance and evaluation standards by September 30, 1994. The amendments also establish a National Commission on Rehabilitation Services to study the quality and adequacy of rehabilitation services provided by the states. After conducting studies and hearings, the National Commission is mandated to submit an interim report by January 30, 1995 and a final report by January 30, 1997.

*Supplementary Security Income* (SSI) is a federal minimum income maintenance program for elders and individuals who are blind or disabled and who meet a test of financial need. Monthly *Social Security Disability Insurance* (SSDI) benefits are available to individuals who are disabled and their dependents, including widowed spouses who are disabled and are 50 years or older (with certain qualifications). To be eligible, individuals must have paid Social Security taxes for a specified number of years (dependent upon the applicant's age); must not be working; and must be declared medically disabled by the state disability determination service or through an appeals process. The disability must be expected to last at least 12 months or to result in death. Individuals who are blind and age 55 to 65 may receive monthly benefits if they are unable to carry out the work (or similar work) that they did before age 55 or becoming blind, whichever is later. Individuals who apply for disability insurance from the Social Security Administration must undergo an evaluation carried out by a state disability evaluation team, composed of physicians, psychologists, and other health care professionals. Social Security disability benefits are not retroactive, so it is important to apply for them immediately after becoming disabled. Social Security disability benefits payments do not begin until six full months after the date that the Social Security office has determined that disability began. At age 65, disability benefits are called retirement benefits even though the dollar amount of benefits remains the same.

The Social Security Administration will provide an estimate of the disability and retirement benefits which any individual has accrued. Since these benefits are based on an average of lifetime earnings under Social Security, it is important to verify that the Social Security Administration has accurate employment records. Women should call the Social Security Administration at (800) 772-1213 to obtain a copy of a "Request for Earnings and Benefit Estimate Statement." Once it is completed and returned, the Social Security Administration will send an estimate of expected benefits. These benefits may be reduced by other government benefits, such as workers' compensation and government pensions.

Women who have received Social Security Disability Insurance for two consecutive years are eligible for *Medicare*, a federal health insurance program which has two parts, hospital insurance and medical insurance. Hospital care and some follow-up care is covered by Medicare Part A. Part B, medical insurance, is paid for by monthly premiums which vary with the type of insurance purchased. Women with low incomes may qualify for a program in which their state pays Medicare premiums and may cover deductibles and coinsurance payments. However, Medicare does not cover eyeglasses (except for recipients who have undergone cataract surgery), low vision aids, or hearing aids. *Medicaid* is a health insurance plan for individuals who are considered financially needy (i.e., recipients of financial benefits from governmental assistance programs, such as Aid to Families with Dependent Children or Supplemental Security Income). Medicaid is a joint federal/state program. While federal law requires that each state cover hospital services, skilled nursing facility services, physician and home health care services, and diagnostic and screening services, states have great discretion in other areas. Payments for prosthetics and rehabilitation equipment vary greatly from state to state.

The medical and social service benefits available from organizations receiving federal assistance are guaranteed by federal laws and protected by the Office of Civil Rights of the Department of Health and Human Services (HHS). When a woman feels that her rights have been violated, a complaint should be filed with the regional office of HHS (see "ORGANIZATIONS" section below).

The *Family and Medical Leave Act* of 1993 (P.L.103-3) requires that employers with 50 or more employees at a worksite or within 75 miles of a worksite must permit eligible employees 12 workweeks of unpaid leave during a 12 month period in order to care for a spouse, son or daughter, or parent who has a serious health condition. During this period of leave, the employer must continue to provide group health benefits for the employee under the same conditions as the employee would have received while working. Upon return from leave, the employee must be restored to the same position s/he had prior to the leave or to a position with equivalent pay, benefits, and conditions of employment. Special regulations apply to employees of school systems and private schools and employees of the federal civil service.

The *Technology-Related Assistance for Individuals with Disabilities Act Amendments of 1994* (P.L. 103-218) strengthens the original Act, passed in 1988. The Act mandates state-wide programs for technology-related assistance to determine needs and resources; to provide technical assistance and information; and to develop demonstration and innovation projects, training programs, and public awareness programs. The amendments set priorities for consumer responsiveness, advocacy, systems change, and outreach to underrepresented populations such as the poor, individuals in rural areas, and minorities.

The *Telecommunications Act of 1996* (P.L. 104-104) requires that manufacturers of telecommunications equipment and providers of telecommunications services ensure that equipment and services are accessible to and usable by individuals with disabilities. If these provisions are not "readily achievable," manufacturers and service providers must ensure that their equipment and services are compatible with the special equipment used by individuals with disabilities to make them accessible. The Architectural and Transportation Barriers Compliance Board (ATBCB) is required to issue guidelines within 18 months of the Act's passage on January 31, 1996.

The *Older Americans Act* (P.L. 89-73) requires that each state office designated to serve elders submit a plan to the Commissioner of the Administration on Aging. This plan must discuss the development of joint programs with the state agency primarily responsible for serving people with disabilities in order to meet the needs of elders with disabilities. The Act also requires that legal services be provided to elders and that each state employ someone to develop legal services to ensure that elders receive these services. Such services could include representing clients in obtaining Social Security benefits and providing legal counseling.

The federal government allows special tax credits for people who are totally disabled and additional standard deductions for those who are legally blind. Legal blindness is defined as acuity of 20/200 or less in the better eye with the best possible correction or a field of 20 degrees or less diameter in the better eye. Tax deductions for business expenses include disability related expenditures, and deductions for medical expenses include special equipment, such as wheelchairs. Contact the Internal Revenue Service (see "ORGANIZATIONS" section below) to obtain publications that explain these benefits, including Publication 501, "Exemptions, Standard Deduction, and Filing Information," and Publication 524, "Credit for the Elderly or the Disabled.".

All states and many local governments have adopted their own laws regarding accessibility. Information about these laws may be obtained from the state or local office serving people with disabilities. In many areas, special legal services for people with disabilities are available, often with fees on a sliding scale. Check with the local bar association or with a law school. Some lawyers specialize in the legal needs of people with disabilities.

The Internet supplies the text of many federal laws and information about federal programs. Individuals who have a connection to the Internet via their university, workplace, or a commercial online service (such as America Online, Delphi, Compuserve, Prodigy, etc.) may search the information available on the Internet by typing "telnet fedworld.gov" and selecting from the menu.

# ORGANIZATIONS

Architectural and Transportation Barriers Compliance Board (ATBCB)
1331 F Street, NW, Suite 1000
Washington, DC 20004-1111
(800) 872-2253                     (800) 993-2822 (TT)                     (202) 272-5434
(202) 272-5449 (TT)                FAX (202) 272-5447
http://www.access-board.gov        BBS (202) 272-5448

A federal agency charged with developing standards for accessibility in federal facilities, public accommodations, and transportation facilities as required by the Americans with Disabilities Act and other federal laws. Provides technical assistance, sponsors research, and distributes publications. Publishes a quarterly newsletter, "Access America." Free. Publications available in standard print, large print, braille, audiocassette, and computer disk.

Clearinghouse on Disability Information
Office of Special Education and Rehabilitative Services (OSERS)
Department of Education
Room 3132, Switzer Building
Washington, DC 20202-2524
(202) 205-8241 (V/TT)              (202) 205-8723 (V/TT)

Responds to inquiries about federal legislation and programs for people with disabilities and makes referrals. Publishes "OSERS Magazine." Free

Commission on Mental and Physical Disability Law
American Bar Association
740 15th Street, NW, 9th Floor
Washington, DC 20005-1009
(202) 662-1570                     (202) 662-1012 (TT)                     FAX (202) 662-1032
e-mail: cmpdl@abanet.org           http://www.abanet.org

Operates a Disability Legal Research Service, which provides searches of databases of laws, legal cases, and recent developments in the field of disability. Provides technical consultations on rights, enforcement, and other issues related to the Americans with Disabilities Act.

Disability Rights Education and Defense Fund (DREDF)
2212 Sixth Street
Berkeley, CA 94710
(510) 644-2555                     (510) 644-2626 (TT)
ADA Hotline: (800) 466-4232 (V/TT), 9:00 am to 5:00 pm, Pacific time
e-mail: dredf.org

Provides technical assistance, information, and referrals on laws and rights; provides legal representation to people with disabilities in both individual and class action cases; trains law students, parents, and legislators. Publishes "Disability Rights News" monthly, available in standard print and audiocassette. Free. ADA Hotline provides information on the Americans with Disabilities Act.

Equal Employment Opportunity Commission (EEOC)
1801 L Street, NW, 10th Floor
Washington, DC 20507
(800) 669-3362 to order publications
(800) 669-4000 to speak to an investigator
(800) 800-3302 (TT)
In the Washington, DC metropolitan area, (202) 275-7377
(202) 275-7518 (TT)                    BBS (202) 514-6193

Responsible for promulgating regulations for the employment section of the ADA. Copies of its regulations are available in standard print, large print, braille, computer disk, and audiocassette. Individuals who feel their employment rights under the ADA have been violated should file a complaint with the EEOC.

Federal Communications Commission (FCC)
1919 M Street, NW
Washington, DC 20554
(202) 418-0190                    (202) 418-2555 (TT)           FAX (202) 418-0232
e-mail: fccinfo@fcc.gov           http://www.fcc.gov

Responsible for developing regulations related to telephone relay services and other requirements of the ADA as it applies to telecommunications.

Internal Revenue Service (IRS)
(800) 829-1040                    (800) 829-4059 (TT)
telnet fedworld.gov               http://www.irs.ustreas.gov

The IRS provides technical assistance about tax credits and deductions related to accommodations for disabilities. To receive Publication 554, "Tax Information for Older Americans," Publication 501, "Exemptions, Standard Deduction, and Filing Information;" Publication 907, "Tax Highlights for Persons with Disabilities;" and Publication 524, "Credit for the Elderly or the Disabled." Call (800) 829-3676; (800) 829-4059 (TT).

National Council on Disability (NCD)
1331 F Street, 10th Floor
Washington, DC 20004
(202) 272-2004                    (202) 272-2074 (TT)           FAX (202) 272-2022

An independent federal agency mandated to study and make recommendations about public policy for people with disabilities. Holds regular meetings and hearings in various locations around the country. Publishes newsletter, "Focus," available in standard print, large print, or on audiocassette. Free

Nolo Self-Help Law Center
Nolo Press
950 Parker Street
Berkeley, CA 94710
(800) 955-4775                    (510) 549-1976                FAX (800) 645-0895
e-mail: noloinfo@nolo.com         http://www.nolo.com

This online service provides information on legal topics, updates legislation and court decisions, and features articles from "Nolo News."

Office of Civil Rights
Department of Education
300 C Street, SW
Washington, DC 20202
(202) 205-5413           (800) 358-8247 (TT)         FAX (202) 205-9862
http://www.ed.gov/offices/OCR

Responsible for enforcing laws and regulations designed to protect the rights of individuals in educational institutions that receive federal financial assistance. Individuals who feel their rights have been violated may file a complaint with one of the ten regional offices located throughout the country.

Office of Civil Rights
Department of Health and Human Services (HHS)
330 Independence Avenue, SW (Cohen Building)
Washington, DC 20201
(202) 619-0585           (202) 863-0101 (TT)         FAX (202) 619-3437
http://www.os.dhhs.gov/progorg/ocr/ocrhmpg.html

Responsible for enforcing laws and regulations that protect the rights of individuals seeking medical and social services in institutions that receive federal financial assistance. Individuals who feel their rights have been violated may file a complaint with one of the ten regional offices located throughout the country.

Office of Federal Contract Compliance Programs (OFCCP)
Department of Labor, Employment Standards Administration
200 Constitution Avenue, NW, Room CC25
Washington, DC 20210
(202) 523-9476           FAX (202) 523-0195
http://www.dol.gov/dol/esa/public/olms_org.htm

Reviews contractors' affirmative action plans, provides technical assistance to contractors, investigates complaints, and resolves issues between contractors and employees. Ten regional offices throughout the country serve as liaisons with the national office and with district offices under their jurisdiction.

Office of Transportation Regulatory Affairs
Department of Transportation
400 Seventh Street, SW
Washington, DC 20590
(202) 366-9305           (202) 755-7687 (TT)

Responsible for promulgating regulations for transportation of individuals with disabilities required by the Rehabilitation Act and the Americans with Disabilities Act. Regulations available in standard print or on audiocassette.

Office on the Americans with Disabilities Act
Department of Justice, Civil Rights Division
PO Box 66118
Washington, DC 20035-6118
(800) 514-0301 Information Line          (800) 514-0383 (TT) Information Line
(202) 514-0301                           (202) 514-0383 (TT)
BBS (202) 514-6193                       http://www.usdoj.gov/crt/ada/adahom1.htm
telnet fedworld.gov

Responsible for enforcing the Americans with Disabilities Act. Copies of its regulations are available in standard print, large print, braille, computer disk, audiocassette, and on the Internet. Callers may request publications, obtain technical assistance, and speak to an ADA specialist.

Social Security Administration
6401 Security Boulevard
Baltimore, MD 21235
(800) 772-1213                           (800) 325-0778 (TT)
http://www.ssa.gov/SSA_Home.html/

To apply for Social Security benefits based on disability, phone the number above to set up an appointment with a Social Security representative, or visit the local Social Security office. Publishes "Social Security Regulations: Rules for Determining Disability and Blindness," free.

Thomas
Library of Congress
http://thomas.loc.gov

This online service provides a database of recent laws and pending legislation, as well as information about the committees of Congress and the text of the "Congressional Record." Searches for legislation and laws may be done by topic or public law number.

# PUBLICATIONS

Americans with Disabilities Act: Questions and Answers
Equal Employment Opportunity Commission (EEOC)
1801 L Street, NW, 10th Floor
Washington, DC 20507
(800) 669-3362 to order publications
In the Washington, DC metropolitan area, (202) 275-7377
(202) 275-7518 (TT)                    FAX (513) 791-2954                    BBS (202) 514-6193

This booklet's question and answer format provides explanations of the ADA's effects on employment, state and local governments, and public accommodations. Large print, audiocassette, braille, and through a bulletin board service. Free

Directory of Legal Aid and Defender Offices
National Legal Aid and Defender Association
1625 K Street, NW, 8th Floor
Washington, DC 20006
(202) 452-0620

A directory of legal aid offices throughout the U.S. Includes chapters on disability protection/advocacy, health law, and senior citizens. Updated biennially. $60.00

Disability Rights and Resources
Demos Vermande
386 Park Avenue South, Suite 201
New York, NY 10016
(800) 532-8663                    (212) 683-0072                    FAX (212) 683-0118

This quarterly newsletter provides information on legal issues, taxes, insurance, and legislation that affect individuals with disabilities and chronic conditions. One year, $19.95; two years, $29.95.

Federal Benefits for Veterans and Dependents
Consumer Information Center
PO Box 100
Pueblo, CO 81002
(719) 948-3334                    BBS (202) 208-7679
e-mail: cic.info@pueblo.gsa.gov     http://www.gsa.gov/staff/pa/cic/cic.htm

This booklet describes the benefits available under federal laws. $3.25

Federal Register
New Orders, Superintendent of Documents
PO Box 371954
Pittsburgh, PA 15250-7954
(202) 512-1800                    FAX (202) 512-2250
telnet federal.bbs.gpo.gov (Port 3001) BBS (202) 512-1661
e-mail: gpoaccess@gpo.gov          http://www.access.gpo.gov/su_docs/aces/desc004.html

A federal publication printed every weekday with notices of all regulations and legal notices issued by federal agencies. Domestic subscriptions, $494.00 annually for second class mailing of paper format; $433.00 annually for microfiche. Free access to the Federal Register is available through the Internet at the address listed above at no charge.

A Guide to Legal Rights for People with Disabilities
by Marc D. Stolman
Demos Vermande
386 Park Avenue South, Suite 201
New York, NY 10016
(800) 532-8663                    (212) 683-0072                    FAX (212) 683-0118

This book discusses civil rights, insurance, benefits, and legal issues faced by individuals with disabilities. Also available on audiocassette and disk (DOS or Mac). $19.95 plus $4.00 shipping and handling.

Life Services Planning for the Elderly and Persons with Disabilities
Commission on Mental and Physical Disability Law
American Bar Association
740 15th Street, NW, 9th Floor
Washington, DC 20005-1009
(202) 662-1570                    (202) 662-1012 (TT)                    FAX (202) 662-1032
e-mail: cmpdl@abanet.org          http://www.abanet.org

This three book series provides guidance for individuals, families, and service providers in estate, financial, health care, and government benefits planning. $20.00 plus $3.95 shipping and handling.

The Medicare Handbook
Social Security Administration
(800) 772-1213                    (800) 325-0778 (TT)
http://www.ssa.gov/SSA_Home.html/

Published annually, this book helps consumers understand their rights under Medicare, including what it pays for, appeal rights, and where to get additional information. Available in English and Spanish, free. Other free publications on Medicare are also available. Also available at local Social Security offices.

Meeting the Needs of Employees with Disabilities
Resources for Rehabilitation
33 Bedford Street, Suite 19A
Lexington, MA 02173
(617) 862-6455                    FAX (617) 861-7517

This book provides information to help people with disabilities retain or obtain employment. Information on government programs and laws, supported employment, training programs, environmental adaptations, and the transition from school to work are included. Chapters on mobility, vision, and hearing and speech impairments include information on organizations, products, and services that enable employers to accommodate the needs of employees with disabilities. $42.95 plus $5.00 shipping and handling. (See order form on last page of this book.)

Mental and Physical Disability Law Reporter
Commission on Mental and Physical Disability Law
American Bar Association
740 15th Street, NW, 9th Floor
Washington, DC 20005-1009
(202) 662-1570                    (202) 662-1012                    FAX (202) 662-1032
e-mail: cmpdl@attmail.com          http://www.abanet.org

A bimonthly journal with court decisions, legislative and regulatory news, and articles on treatment, accessibility, employment, education, federal programs, etc. Individuals, $229.00; organizations, $289.00. Reprints of articles from back issues available.

Pocket Guide to Federal Help for Individuals with Disabilities
Clearinghouse on Disability Information
Office of Special Education and Rehabilitative Services (OSERS)
Room 3132, Switzer Building
Washington, DC 20202-2524
(202) 205-8241 (V/TT)             (202) 205-8723 (V/TT)

A summary of benefits and services available from the federal government. Free

Red Book on Work Incentives
A Summary Guide to Social Security and Supplemental Security Income Work Incentives for People with Disabilities
Social Security Administration
(800) 772-1213                    (800) 325-0778 (TT)
http://www.ssa.gov/SSA_Home.html/

Overview of work incentives for individuals who receive SSDI or SSI. Includes impairment-related work expenses, trial work period, continuation of Medicare coverage, earned income exclusion, and other work incentives. Also available from local Social Security offices. Large print, free.

Regulation, Litigation and Dispute Resolution Under the Americans with Disabilities Act: A Practitioner's Guide to Implementation
Commission on Mental and Physical Disability Law
American Bar Association
740 15th Street, NW, 9th Floor
Washington, DC 20005-1009
(202) 662-1570                    (202) 662-1012 (TT)                FAX (202) 662-1032
e-mail: cmpdl@abanet.org          http://www.abanet.org

An analysis of the law, with emphasis on government services, employment, housing, health insurance, and public accommodations. $35.00 plus $4.95 shipping and handling.

Report on Disability Programs
Business Publishers
951 Pershing Drive
Silver Spring, MD 20910
(800) 274-0122                    (301) 587-6300                    FAX (301) 585-9075
http://www.bpinews.com

A biweekly newsletter with information on policies promulgated by federal agencies, laws, and funding sources.  $297.00

A Summary of Department of Veterans Affairs Benefits
(800) 827-1000

This booklet is available from any VA regional office.  Free

Summary of Existing Legislation Affecting Persons with Disabilities
Office of Special Education and Rehabilitative Services (OSERS)
Clearinghouse on Disability Information
Room 3132, Switzer Building
Washington, DC 20202-2524
(202) 205-8241 (V/TT)                    (202) 205-8723 (V/TT)

This book includes the legislative history and major provisions of laws related to income maintenance programs, health, education, housing, social services, vocational rehabilitation, and transportation. Free

Tax Options and Strategies: A State-by-State Guide for Persons with Disabilities, Senior Citizens, Veterans, and Their Families
by Bruce E. Bondo
Demos Vermande
386 Park Avenue South, Suite 201
New York, NY 10016
(800) 532-8663                    (212) 683-0072                    FAX (212) 683-0118

This book provides information that enables individuals to benefit from federal, state, and local tax provisions such as tax exemptions, credits, and deductions.  $24.95 plus $4.00 shipping and handling.

Tax Options and Strategies for People with Disabilities
by Steven Mendelsohn
Demos Vermande
386 Park Avenue South, Suite 201
New York, NY 10016
(800) 532-8663                    (212) 683-0072                    FAX (212) 683-0118

This book describes provisions in the tax laws that affect individuals with disabilities, including access to retirement funds to defray disability related expenses, deductions available for assistive technology, incentives for employers to hire individuals with disabilities, and dependent care.  Also available on audiocassette and disk (DOS or Mac).  $24.95 plus $4.00 shipping and handling.

<u>Understanding Social Security</u>
<u>Working While Disabled... How Social Security Can Help</u>
Social Security Administration
(800) 772-1213                              (800) 325-0778 (TT)
http://www.ssa.gov/SSA_Home.html/

These booklets provide basic information about Social Security programs. The Social Security Administration distributes many other titles, including "Disability," "Medicare," "Retirement," "SSI," and "Survivors." Many of these titles are available in large print, braille, or audiocassette. Also available at local Social Security offices, free.

<u>The Women's Legal Defense Fund's Guide to Using the Family and Medical Leave Act: Questions and Answers</u>
Women's Legal Defense Fund
1875 Connecticut Avenue, NW, Suite 710
Washington, DC 20009
(202) 986-2600                              FAX (202) 986-2539

This booklet answers the most frequently asked questions about the law. $10.00

# Chapter 4

# *ARTHRITIS*

Although rheumatoid arthritis and osteoarthritis are two common rheumatic diseases found in women, the conditions develop at different stages of life and have different symptoms. Some women may have both conditions. Since osteoarthritis usually affects women later in life, it is described below in the section titled "Arthritis in Older Women."

Rheumatoid arthritis is a chronic, systemic, inflammatory disease that can affect the entire body but is most commonly found in the hands, wrists, and feet. It occurs three times more frequently in women than in men. Over five million American women 15 years old and over reported arthritis and rheumatism as the cause of limitations in physical activities and activities of daily living, the most prevalent condition causing limitations for women (McNeil: 1993). The disease affects the synovium, which is the membrane that lines the joints and provides them with nourishment and lubrication. Rheumatoid arthritis causes the synovium to become inflamed (synovitis), swollen, and painful. Eventually the bone cartilage is affected, causing pain and further damaging joints. Fatigue, depression, weight loss, and anemia are common. Rheumatoid arthritis may also cause inflammation in other body organs, affecting the blood vessels and the outer lining of the heart and lungs. Although rheumatoid arthritis can occur in children (juvenile rheumatoid arthritis), onset peaks between the ages of 20 and 50 (Arthritis Foundation: 1994a). Eighty percent of the women who develop rheumatoid arthritis are between the ages of 35 and 50 (Lipsky: 1994). Some researchers have linked an inherited tendency to develop rheumatoid arthritis with genetic markers controlling immune system function, while others suspect that infections trigger the development of rheumatoid arthritis (Arthritis Foundation: 1994a).

Rheumatoid arthritis subsides and flares unpredictably, causes severe pain, and may lead to substantial or complete disability. In contrast to many other forms of arthritis, rheumatoid arthritis develops symmetrically, affecting the same joint on both sides of the body (knees, wrists, knuckles, etc.). The stages of functional incapacity include normal activity with no restrictions; adequate function with some pain and moderate restrictions; limited ability to work or to provide self care; confinement to bed; or requiring the use of a wheelchair (Bennett: 1988).

Diagnosing rheumatoid arthritis is difficult. Many individuals describe their condition as "flu-like," citing muscle aches and fatigue. Since symptoms vary among individuals, other rheumatic diseases may be considered initially. Blood tests and x-rays are commonly used, as well as criteria established by the American College of Rheumatology. These criteria include joint swelling and pain for more than six weeks, marked joint and muscle stiffness in the morning, evidence of bone damage, nodules characteristic of rheumatoid arthritis under the skin, and the presence of a rheumatoid antibody in the blood. This antibody, called a rheumatoid factor, is found in 80 to 90% of individuals diagnosed with rheumatoid arthritis (Shlotzhauer and McGuire: 1993). About a fifth of the individuals with rheumatoid arthritis develop pea sized nodules under the skin, which are actually inflamed blood vessels. These nodules appear sporadically during the course of the disease. Although they rarely cause problems, they are indicative of an acute form of the disease.

Some individuals with rheumatoid arthritis develop a related rheumatic condition known as Sjogren's syndrome, which affects the tear, salivary, and other moisture producing glands. Corneal erosions, conjunctivitis, and inflammation of the front of the eye are complications of the lack of tears. Sjogren's syndrome is ten times more frequent in women than in men (American College of Rheumatology: no date). Treatment options include artificial tears and ointments or pellets placed between the eyelid and eyeball that dissolve slowly, releasing moisture to the eye.

Multipurpose Arthritis and Musculoskeletal Diseases Centers, created by the National Arthritis Act of 1975, have been established across the United States. Fourteen centers are currently investigating the roles of physiological treatment and psychosocial interventions in the care of individuals with rheumatic diseases (Freeman et al.: 1996).

## *TREATMENT*

Early diagnosis and treatment are key to the prevention of the deformities of the joints often associated with rheumatoid arthritis. Treatment aims to prevent joint destruction through the use of medication that reduces joint inflammation and relieves pain, rest, and exercise to restore and protect joint and muscle function. Women who fear disability due to arthritis may delay seeking treatment, placing themselves at greater risk for potential damage. Pain is the major manifestation of arthritis; therefore, pain management should be a prime concern for both women and their health care providers.

For many years, nonsteroidal anti-inflammatory drugs (NSAIDs) such as aspirin have been the most common medications used to treat arthritis, because they reduce joint inflammation and pain. Side effects of treatment with NSAIDs include stomach irritation, constipation, nausea, fluid retention, dizziness, and blood clotting problems. According to the Arthritis Foundation (1996), being female confers a greater risk of developing an ulcer while taking NSAIDs. Additional ulcer risk factors are age (over 60), a history of ulcers, use of corticosteroids, the presence of another chronic disease, drinking alcohol, and smoking. NSAIDs such as ibuprofen and naproxen are similar to aspirin but may have fewer side effects, although they have been implicated in gastrointestinal bleeding and renal problems (Fenner: 1992). Other drugs which may be used are antimalarial drugs, gold salts, steroids (prednisone, cortisone, and others), methotrexate, and penicillamine (not the same as penicillin) (U.S. Department of Health and Human Services: 1982). On rare occasions, antimalarial drugs cause damage to the retina of the eye, a side effect that is usually reversible (Fries: 1995). Because of the possibility of this side effect, women should see an ophthalmologist for eye examinations before and during the course of treatment with antimalarials. Steroids may accelerate the development of osteoporosis and affect diabetes and blood pressure. Because of the many and serious potential side effects of these drugs, a woman should be certain to obtain all possible information about contraindications, probability of side effects, and permanency of side effects before making the decision to take these medications.

Currently there is controversy even within the medical community regarding the classic treatment plan for rheumatoid arthritis, referred to as the "pyramid" treatment plan. In this plan aspirin and other NSAIDs form the base of the pyramid; the next drug choices are antimalarials and gold salts; then methotrexate, penicillamine, and azathioprine; and, at the top of the pyramid, cytotoxins and other powerful immunosuppressive drugs (Arthritis Foundation: 1991). Some rheumatologists believe that the risk of potential toxic effects is outweighed by the opportunity to prevent joint destruction by treating active disease aggressively. Others believe that more powerful drugs should be prescribed only when the least toxic drugs no longer control inflammation, prevent joint damage, or enable easy movement. The Arthritis Foundation (1994a) reports that methotrexate has been shown to maintain control of the disease over periods of more than five years in a larger proportion of people with rheumatoid arthritis than those treated with other medications, such as gold salts. A meta-analysis of data from multiple clinical trials concluded that methotrexate and antimalarials provided maximum efficacy with the least toxicity (Freeman et al.: 1996). Women who take methotrexate are monitored carefully for liver function and white blood cell counts. Contraindications for methotrexate therapy include kidney, lung, and heart disease. Abstention from drinking alcohol during methotrexate treatment is advised.

If medication and physical therapy are insufficient for pain management and there is evidence of joint damage, orthopedic surgery may be required, such as knee, hip, shoulder, and wrist arthroplasty (total replacement), or arthrodesis (joint fusion). Prosthetic joints may wear out, and the risk of infection requires careful medical monitoring over time. Since multiple joint damage is common in individuals with rheumatoid arthritis, it is crucial to evaluate functional capacities before surgery. For example, will a woman undergoing a knee replacement be able to use crutches during the recuperative period? If wrist, elbow, or shoulder joints are painful, how will she ambulate with crutches? Women treated with corticosteroids are more susceptible to infection and thinning of the skin. Aspirin treatment may interfere with blood clotting factors and should be discontinued at least a week before surgery to avoid bleeding during surgery and postoperatively. Individuals contemplating surgery must also be evaluated for their ability and motivation to participate in a long postoperative rehabilitation program.

The role of exercise in increasing endurance for women with arthritis is currently receiving increased attention. Jurisson (1991) reports that a decrease in symptoms is an unexpected benefit of exercises, such as walking, aquatics, and riding a stationary bicycle. Individuals with arthritis benefit from a daily routine combining strengthening, range of motion, and endurance exercises followed by rest and relaxation.

A program of physical therapy may include heat and cold treatments, massage, and relaxation training. Heat treatments may include hot baths or showers, hot packs, heat lamps, electric pads or mitts, paraffin wax applications, or blown hot air. Cold compresses or ice bags may also be effective. Transcutaneous electrical nerve stimulation (TENS) may be used to relieve pain. The physical therapist may recommend the use of canes, walkers, or crutches to reduce the body's weight on joints. Physical therapists may also provide instruction in using the joints more safely; for example, pushing with the whole arm or side of the body rather than with the hand only. Splints or orthotics, which are devices used for support and to improve function in movable parts of the body, may be prescribed to stabilize weak joints and prevent them from becoming permanently stiff or bent. The physical therapist may also recommend rest to relieve inflammation and pain, although too much rest may lead to stiffness and poor joint movement. It is necessary to achieve a balance between rest during flares and activity during remissions.

## ARTHRITIS IN OLDER WOMEN

Osteoarthritis, the most common type of arthritis in older women, is a chronic, nonsystemic, noninflammatory form of arthritis which results in the breakdown of the cartilage that covers the ends of the bones and other joint tissue. Age is a major risk factor in the development of osteoarthritis, and it is more common in women over the age of 54 than men (Arthritis Foundation: 1994b). An x-ray survey of women revealed that while 30% of women ages 45 to 64 showed evidence of osteoarthritis, 68% of women over age 65 had developed the condition (Brandt: 1994).

Osteoarthritis does not affect the entire body but most commonly occurs in the joints of the fingers, hips, and knees, and the discs of the spine. It is a degenerative disease, formerly thought to be related to the overuse and abuse of joints through the "wear and tear" of aging. Actually, activity seems to protect joints. Lorig and Fries (1990) report that studies of individuals engaged in activities that put stress on joints, such as long distance runners and those who operate pneumatic drills, are at no greater risk for osteoarthritis. Obesity is a far greater risk factor for osteoarthritis of the knee. The Arthritis Foundation (1994b) reports that controlling or losing weight may reduce this risk, citing a study in which women who lost as little as 11 pounds over a ten year span halved their risk for osteoarthritis of the knee.

The most common signs of osteoarthritis are painful bony growths in the joints of the fingers. Osteoarthritis may also occur in a single joint due to injury or infection. Sports injuries, for example, may increase the risk of developing osteoarthritis. Osteoarthritis develops gradually, resulting in mild to severe disability. A woman's medical history and findings from a physical examination are often sufficient to suspect that she has osteoarthritis. X-rays, which detect the growth of bony spurs or the narrowing of space between joints due to wearing away of cartilage, are used to confirm a diagnosis of osteoarthritis.

The most common medications used to treat osteoarthritis by reducing pain are analgesics and nonsteroidal anti-inflammatory drugs (NSAIDs). Researchers who have compared these two options found that there was no difference in the relief of symptoms, although NSAIDS are more expensive and have greater risk of side effects (Brandt: 1993). It is recommended that these drugs be taken with meals in order to reduce stomach irritation.

Range of motion exercises strengthen joints and reduce the loss of physical functioning. Walking and swimming help women maintain flexible joints and also provide aerobic exercise that is good for the entire body and the sense of well-being. Swimming is particularly good for women whose knees and hips are affected. Exercise in the water reduces the stress on these major joints while increasing cardiovascular health and endurance.

Severe osteoarthritis in the hip may require total hip replacement surgery, to restore function and relieve pain. Since total hip replacements last an average of 15 years (Lorig and Fries: 1990), it is important to think about facing the pain, risk, and costs of repeating the procedure. It is wise to participate in a rehabilitation program following this surgery. Physical and occupational therapy services may be provided at a rehabilitation center, outpatient clinic, or in the home. Knee replacement surgery has become more common and successful in recent years. Maintaining a healthy weight and exercising daily will contribute to postsurgical success. Older women should investigate the benefits of joint replacement surgery very carefully, seeking more than one opinion, and taking their time in making a decision.

## SEXUAL FUNCTIONING

The woman coping with rheumatoid arthritis may experience problems with sexual functioning, becoming self-conscious about body image due to weight gain associated with use of steroid drugs. In addition, she may experience deformed joints; fatigue; and lack of energy. A loss of self-esteem commonly occurs. Some women may avoid sexual relations, fearing pain or rejection. Depression, resulting from chronic arthritic pain, may also cause decreased interest in sexual activity (Ehrlich: 1973). A partner who fears causing pain may hesitate to initiate sexual relations, reinforcing the woman's feeling of rejection. If neither partner is willing to discuss these feelings, relationships suffer. Communication between partners is key to living with a chronic disease as well as to maintaining sexual function.

Vaginal dryness, a complication often experienced by women with rheumatoid arthritis (Fries: 1995), may cause painful intercourse. A commercial, water soluble lubricant may alleviate this problem. However, once the woman has experienced pain during intercourse, she may avoid future sexual encounters because of her fears. Medications prescribed to reduce pain may also reduce libido. Anti-inflammatory medication should be scheduled so that it will provide maximum relief during sexual relations. Fatigue and a diminished range of motion may also affect sexual function. A warm bath or shower may help to relax joints and muscles. A water bed or flotation mattress may make movement less painful and reduce stress on joints. Experimenting with new positions for intercourse that put less stress on the affected joints may be helpful. Placing a pillow under the hips or wearing

110

knee pads may relieve stress on these joints. Regular exercise may help reduce weakness, contribute to weight control, and increase feelings of well-being.

## FAMILY PLANNING, PREGNANCY, AND CHILDREARING

Women who do not wish to become pregnant should choose contraceptive methods with care. Birth control pills are reliable and may be preferable for women whose manual dexterity makes barrier methods difficult to use.

Since rheumatoid arthritis affects women of childbearing age, couples must weigh the decision to have children carefully. They must evaluate the risk to both mother and fetus, the effects of treatment, and the effects on the family. Medications may affect fertility in the woman experiencing a flare. It is a good idea to seek obstetric care from a physician with experience in the management of high risk pregnancies who will work with the rheumatologist to provide the best possible care.

Although it is safe to continue taking most arthritis medications during pregnancy, it is important to discuss their use with both rheumatologist and obstetrician. Weinblatt (1993) suggests that women wishing to conceive should discontinue treatment with methotrexate for at least one menstrual cycle prior to attempting conception. The Arthritis Foundation (1994a) recommends that methotrexate be discontinued several months prior to a planned pregnancy and throughout the course of pregnancy in order to prevent birth defects. Nor should methotrexate be taken when breastfeeding. Immunosuppressive drugs should be continued during pregnancy only if the mother's health is at serious risk (Kean and Buchanan: 1990). Salicylates, such as aspirin, should be discontinued several weeks before the due date to avoid blood clotting problems and anemia in the mother. Salicylates should not be taken after delivery if the mother is breastfeeding, because they are excreted in breast milk. It is recommended that NSAIDs be prescribed at the lowest possible dose during the first four months of gestation. They, too, are excreted in breast milk and should be discontinued while the mother is nursing her baby. Corticosteroids, injected into affected joints rather than taken orally, may be used to control inflammation with little effect on the fetus. Cases of nerve deafness in the infant caused by antimalarials have also been reported (Klipple and Cecere: 1989).

Generally, women with rheumatoid arthritis deliver their babies with no complications. However, women with hip deformities who cannot spread their legs wide enough for a vaginal delivery will require a cesarean delivery (Rogers and Matsumura: 1991). Cervical spine x-rays, taken before conception, will show potential problems if intubation is necessary for the administration of anesthesia. Regional anesthesia, such as an epidural, may be preferred for delivery if there is any evidence of cervical subluxation (slippage of the joints).

Klipple and Cecere (1989) report that 70% of women with rheumatoid arthritis experience some remission of their symptoms while pregnant and that subsequent pregnancies also follow this course. Remission of rheumatoid arthritis symptoms will most likely end after the baby's birth, returning the mother to her pre-pregnancy status. More than 90% of the women in one of their studies experienced a relapse within six to eight months after delivery.

The pregnant woman with rheumatoid arthritis should develop a schedule that allows for rest periods during the day, eight to ten hours of sleep per night, and the opportunity to sit down for rest frequently during the course of the day. She should continue the exercise routine she followed prior to pregnancy and may find that swimming provides an ideal workout, protecting weight-bearing joints from the stress of weight gain associated with pregnancy. A woman may need assistance during the period of adjustment to motherhood, especially if a probable flare of symptoms occurs. Siblings may resent the new baby not only for the attention being paid to their new sister or brother, but also because their mother's symptoms have flared and she is exhausted and in pain.

Couples should consider the potential for stress on the partner due to the extra duties necessitated by the mothers's fatigue during pregnancy. Increased fatigue, stiffness, and pain after delivery; and a possible combination of postpartum depression with disappointment at the return of rheumatic disease activity are potential problems for the mother. Financial matters may be an issue if the couple is dependent on the wife's earnings and she is unable to return to work. The physical duties of baby care, such as lifting, bathing, and carrying the infant, must be planned in advance in the event the disease flares after delivery.

Women with rheumatoid arthritis may find that maternity and baby clothes need adaptations for easier use. Maternity clothes can be adapted with velcro closures. Bending over to tie shoes can be avoided when elastic shoelaces are substituted for conventional laces. Maternity or nursing brassieres with front hooks or velcro fasteners eliminate the problem of fastening hooks in the rear. A baby sling relieves the strain of carrying the infant. A nursing pillow used to support the baby and a breast pump operated by foot are useful when breastfeeding (see Chapter 2, "VENDORS OF ASSISTIVE DEVICES," page 81). When the child is sick, an ear thermometer which is larger and therefore easier to hold may be substituted for a conventional thermometer; large medicine droppers or a bottle may be used to give medications.

Women with arthritis face additional challenges in childrearing. Not only must they cope with the responsibilities of home and family, but often they must cope with pain and lack of energy too. It is difficult for children to understand when a parent cannot attend a sports event or prepare refreshments for a school activity due to an arthritis flare. Young children sometimes think that a mother's illness is in some way their fault. Children also fear that they, too, will develop the condition. If mothers find it difficult to discuss a chronic condition with their children, it may be helpful for the family to work with a social worker, physical therapist, or other health professional. Many support groups invite families to attend their meetings in order to provide them with emotional support and practical information. The group setting may help family members understand functional losses as well as fatigue and pain of arthritis. Providing respite care for women with arthritis and their families in the form of babysitting and cleaning services may prove to be extremely valuable.

## PSYCHOLOGICAL ASPECTS OF ARTHRITIS

Women with arthritis must learn how to adjust to the flares and remissions associated with their particular condition; to cope with pain; and to determine the best medical treatment for their specific needs. Arthritis is often a "hidden" disease, since symptoms such as fatigue and morning stiffness are unpredictable. When the symptoms are active, the woman may be in obvious pain; when rested or when treatment reduces pain, it is hard for others to understand her limitations. It is important for the physician to explain these aspects of arthritis.

When arthritis makes work and activities of daily living difficult, it may affect interpersonal relationships both on the job and at home. If the woman is tired, in pain, or unable to move about easily, she may experience emotional problems, such as depression, loss of self-esteem, and worry, which in turn make everyday life even more difficult. These problems combined with mood changes due to medication may also lead to sexual dysfunction (Gerber: 1988). The Arthritis Foundation recommends learning stress reduction or relaxation techniques and participating in recreational activities and social groups.

Arthritis also affects the dual roles of women as workers outside the home and homemakers. Allaire (1992) reports that little role disability is encountered by women with mild arthritis, but that women with more severe disease are likely to have both employment and household disability. Allaire (1992) recommends that rehabilitation interventions address both employment and homemaker goals.

Her subjects with severe disease activity tried to maintain their roles as homemakers through a combination of adaptive aids, help from partners and children, and changing their standards for household tasks, such as cleaning and meal preparation. A study of gender differences in osteoarthritis suggests that caregiving responsibilities may delay a woman's decision to undergo knee or hip replacement surgery (Freeman et al.: 1996).

## *PROFESSIONAL SERVICE PROVIDERS*

Services for women with arthritis are provided by a variety of health care professionals. In addition, voluntary organizations provide information, education, and support groups.

*Internists* or *family physicians*, who provide primary care, may diagnose and approve treatment for rheumatoid arthritis. Often they refer individuals to a rheumatologist for confirmation of the diagnosis and with whom they will coordinate treatment. *Rheumatologists* are physicians who specialize in the treatment of rheumatic diseases, which are inflammations and degenerations of joints and connective tissues. Rheumatologists may serve as case coordinators for women who receive treatment from a multidisciplinary team. *Orthopedic surgeons* or *plastic surgeons* may perform surgery to repair or replace joints damaged by arthritis. *Physiatrists* are physicians who specialize in rehabilitation medicine, often arranging for treatment from physical and occupational therapists.

*Obstetricians* are physicians who provide primary care during pregnancy, labor and delivery, and postpartum. Some may be specialists in treating women with high risk pregnancies due to chronic disease; they should work with rheumatologists to provide multidisciplinary care during pregnancy.

*Physical therapists* develop an exercise program to control some arthritic symptoms; keep joints flexible; build up and preserve muscle strength; and help protect joints from further stress. *Occupational therapists* teach new techniques to perform everyday activities, such as washing and dressing, homemaking, and recreation. They may make suggestions regarding safety and sources of assistive devices, such as reaching tools, built-up kitchen utensils, and writing aids.

*Social workers* provide information about financial and medical benefits, housing, and community resources. They conduct individual, family, or group counseling and may refer individuals to self-help or peer counseling groups.

*Rehabilitation counselors* help individuals with arthritis develop a plan that will enable them to continue functioning and working. Some individuals will need assistance in returning to their previous position or retraining to obtain a different type of position. Rehabilitation counselors help make the contacts and placements necessary to attain these goals.

## *WHERE TO FIND SERVICES*

The health care professionals who provide services to women with rheumatoid arthritis and osteoarthritis work in hospitals, rehabilitation centers, home health agencies, private and public agencies, independent living centers, and as private practitioners. Individual and group counseling may be available through a local hospital, community health center, senior center, or from mental health professionals in private practice. Patient education programs are offered by hospitals, universities, and chapters of both the Arthritis Foundation in the United States and the Arthritis Society in Canada in order to help individuals live as independently as possible. These courses often result in reduction in pain, dependency, and depression (National Resource Center on Health Promotion and Aging: 1989). Common topics in these courses are education about arthritis, exercise, emotional support, and discussions of how individuals can advocate for themselves within the health care system and participate in choosing treatment options. The Arthritis Foundation offers a six week self-help course, which has been found to increase participants' perception of their own control over the disease, which in turn improves their health status (Haggerty: 1995). Exercise programs in heated pools are also sponsored by local chapters of the Arthritis Foundation. Some women attend pain clinics which teach behavior modification techniques to control the effect of pain.

Women who are severely disabled by arthritis often require home health services. These services are provided by nurses or home health aides; special homemaker services; Meals on Wheels programs; chore services such as housecleaning; and adult day activity programs. The services are often free to individuals with low incomes, or the fees may be on a sliding scale.

Women with rheumatoid arthritis or osteoarthritis require hospitalization when joint replacement surgery is necessary. After surgery, they may move to a rehabilitation unit within the hospital where the surgery was performed or to a rehabilitation hospital. Most rehabilitation centers also offer out-patient services.

## ASSISTIVE DEVICES AND ENVIRONMENTAL ADAPTATIONS

Many individuals with arthritis use assistive devices to make everyday living easier. These devices may be specially designed, or they may be common items found in medical supply or hardware stores. They may be purchased in local stores or through mail order catalogues. Schweidler (1984) identifies four basic functions of assistive devices for people with arthritis: to compensate for lost function; to alleviate joint stress; to decrease energy demands; and to increase safety.

The physical therapist or occupational therapist may recommend using an assistive device only at times when functioning is difficult. Women with arthritis must keep their joints flexible yet protect them from stress. It is also important to learn to use the assistive device correctly to avoid stress on other joints.

Devices such as can and jar openers compensate for a weak grasp. Long-handled tongs, utensils with built-up handles, and other adapted equipment will make it easier to continue homemaking activities. Special lamps are controlled with a pat of the hand. A pen with a thick barrel is easier to use than a slim design, because it reduces stress on finger joints. Dressing aids, such as button hooks, elastic shoe laces, a long-handled shoe horn, sock-aid, or zipper pulls, and clothing with velcro fasteners, elastic waistbands, or snaps enable a woman to conserve energy when dressing. Reachers may be used to pick up items that have fallen to the floor or to reach items in overhead cabinets. It is easier to open and close doors when doorknobs are replaced with levers, push locks, or push-pull latches. Swing clear hinges on doors provide the clearance to accommodate wheelchairs and walkers, which some women with arthritis use in order to ambulate. Adjustable height sinks and toilets are valuable additions in the bathroom as are grab bars, long-handled bath brushes, and bath benches for safety in the tub or shower. A cane may make walking safer by promoting balance. Battery powered chairs help individuals who cannot walk long distances or stand for long periods of time continue activities, such as visiting museums and attending sports events. Assistive devices for recreational activities include cardholders, bookstands, and adapted gardening tools that reduce bending and ease grasping.

An automobile with power steering, brakes, windows and seat controls reduces stress on joints. General Motors, Ford, Saturn, and Chrysler offer financial assistance for the purchase of adaptive equipment such as hand controls, a ramp, or lifts to be installed in vehicles (see Chapter 2, "ORGANIZATIONS," page 85). Special van services or special parking placards for individuals with arthritis may help solve some transportation problems. Architectural adaptations such as ramps, railings, chairlifts, and elevators may make independent mobility easier.

Although most assistive devices are nonprescription items, some may be covered by third-party payment with prior approval.

References

Allaire, Saralynn H.
1992    "Employment and Household Work Disability in Women with Rheumatoid Arthritis" <u>Journal of Applied Rehabilitation Counseling</u> 23:1:44-51

American College of Rheumatology
No date    <u>Fact Sheet: Sjogren's Syndrome</u> Atlanta, GA: American College of Rheumatology

Arthritis Foundation
1996    <u>Aspirin and Other NSAIDS</u> Atlanta, GA: The Arthritis Foundation
1994a    <u>Rheumatoid Arthritis</u> Atlanta, GA: The Arthritis Foundation
1994b    <u>Osteoarthritis</u>  Atlanta, GA: The Arthritis Foundation
1991    "Effective RA Drug Treatment: Changing the Strategy?" <u>Joint Movement</u> 2:2:1-3

Bennett, J. Claude
1988    "Clinical Features" pp. 87-92 in H. Ralph Schumacher, Jr. (ed.) <u>Primer on the Rheumatic Diseases</u> Atlanta, GA: Arthritis Foundation

Brandt, Kenneth D.
1994    "Osteoarthritis" pp. 1692-1698 in Kurt J. Isselbacher et al. (eds.) <u>Harrison's Principles of Internal Medicine</u> New York, NY: McGraw Hill
1993    "NSAIDs in the Treatment of Osteoarthritis:  Friends or Foes?" <u>Bulletin on the Rheumatic Diseases</u> 42:6:1-4

Ehrlich, George E.
1973    <u>Total Management of the Arthritic Patient</u> Philadelphia, PA: J.B. Lippincott Company

Fenner, Helmut
1992    "Nonsteroidal Anti-inflammatory Drugs: Benefit/Risk Evaluation in Rheumatic Diseases" <u>Journal of Rheumatology</u> 19:(Supplement 32):98-99

Freeman, Julia B. et al.
1996    "Advances Brought by Health Services Research to Patients with Arthritis: Summary of the Workshop on Health Services Research in Arthritis: From Research to Practice" <u>Arthritis Care and Research</u> 9 (April):2:142-150

Fries, James F.
1995    <u>Arthritis:  A Take Care of Yourself Health Guide</u> Reading, MA: Addison-Wesley-Longman Publishing Company

Gerber, Lynn H.
1988    "Rehabilitative Therapies for Patients with Rheumatic Disease" pp. 301-307 in H. Ralph Schumacher, Jr. (ed.) <u>Primer on the Rheumatic Diseases</u> Atlanta, GA: Arthritis Foundation

Haggerty, Maureen
1995    "Taking Control" <u>Advance/Rehabilitation</u> 4(January)6:35-38

Jurisson, Mary L.
1991    "Rehabilitation in Rheumatic Diseases  What's New" <u>Western Journal of Medicine</u> 154:5:545-548

Kean, W.F. and W.W. Buchanan
1990    "Pregnancy and Rheumatoid Arthritis" <u>Baillieres Clinical Rheumatology</u> 4(1):125-40

Klipple, Gary L. and Fred A. Cecere
1989    "Rheumatoid Arthritis and Pregnancy" <u>Rheumatic Disease Clinics of North America</u> 15:2:213-239

Lipsky, Peter E.

1994    "Rheumatoid Arthritis" pp. 1648-1655 in Isselbacher, Kurt J. et al. (eds.) <u>Harrison's Principles of Internal Medicine</u> New York, NY: McGraw Hill

Lorig, Kate and James F. Fries

1990    <u>The Arthritis Helpbook</u> Reading, MA: Addison-Wesley Publishing Company

McNeil, John M.

1993    <u>Americans with Disabilities: 1991-92</u> U.S. Bureau of the Census, Current Population Reports, P70-33 Washington, DC: U.S. Government Printing Office

National Resource Center on Health Promotion and Aging

1989    "Arthritis: Positive Approaches Offer New Hope" <u>Perspectives in Health Promotion and Aging</u> 4:(November-December)6

Rogers, Judith and Molleen Matsumura

1991    <u>Mother-to-Be: A Guide to Pregnancy and Birth for Women with Disabilities</u> New York, NY: Demos Publications

Schweidler, Helen

1984    "Assistive Devices, Aids to Daily Living" pp. 263-276 in Gail Kershner Riggs and Eric P. Gall (eds.) <u>Rheumatic Diseases, Rehabilitation and Management</u> Boston, MA: Butterworth

Shlotzhauer, Tammi L. and James L. McGuire

1993    <u>Living with Rheumatoid Arthritis</u> Baltimore, MD: Johns Hopkins University Press

U.S. Department of Health and Human Services

1982    "Arthritis Advice" <u>Age Page</u> Washington, DC: National Institute on Aging

Weinblatt, Michael E.

1993    "Methotrexate in Rheumatoid Arthritis" <u>Bulletin on the Rheumatic Diseases</u> 42:4:4-7 Atlanta, GA: The Arthritis Foundation

# ORGANIZATIONS

American College of Rheumatology
60 Executive Park South, Suite 150
Atlanta, GA 30329
(404) 633-3777                     FAX (404) 633-1870
http://www.rheumatology.org

A professional membership organization for rheumatologists who treat or study all forms of arthritis. Will provide a state-by-state list of rheumatologists.

Arthritis Foundation
1314 Spring Street, NW
Atlanta, GA 30309
(800) 283-7800            (404) 872-7100            FAX (404) 872-0457
http://www@arthritis.org

Supports research; offers referrals to rheumatologists; provides public and professional education; sponsors arthritis classes and clubs, exercise programs, and discount drug services. Chapters and divisions across the U.S. Membership, $20.00, includes chapter newsletter and bimonthly magazine, "Arthritis Today."

Arthritis Society
250 Bloor Street East, Suite 901
Toronto, Ontario M4W 3P2 Canada
(416) 967-1414            FAX (416) 967-7171
http://www.arthritis.ca

Supports research on the causes and cures for arthritis and medical training programs; provides information and educational materials; establishes self-help groups; and in some provinces, administers pool-therapy and home-visit programs. Division offices in every province. Publishes "Arthritis News" and "Communique" (in French), quarterly. Subscription, $10.00, Canadian funds.

National Arthritis and Musculoskeletal and Skin Diseases Information Clearinghouse
1 AMS Circle
Bethesda, MD 20892-3675
(301) 495-4484            (301) 565-2966 (TT)            FAX (301) 587-4352

Compiles and distributes information to health care professionals through a database. Distributes bibliographies, fact sheets, catalogues, and directories. Requests from individuals are referred to the Arthritis Foundation.

National Institute of Arthritis and Musculoskeletal and Skin Diseases (NIAMS)
Building 31, Room 4C-32
9000 Rockville Pike
Bethesda, MD 20892
(301) 496-8190            FAX (301) 480-6069            http://www.nih.gov/niams

NIAMS supports Multi-Purpose Arthritis Centers, which conduct basic and clinical research; provide professional, public, and patient education; and sponsor community activities.

National Sjogren's Syndrome Association
PO Box 42207
Phoenix, AZ 85080-2207
(800) 395-6772                    (602) 516-0787                    FAX (602) 516-0111
e-mail: NSSA@aol.com

Provides information to individuals and professionals through support groups and conferences throughout the U.S.  Membership, $25.00, includes quarterly "Patient Education Series" and newsletter, "Sjogren's Digest."

Sjogren's Syndrome Foundation
333 North Broadway
Jericho, NY 11753
(800) 475-6473                    (516) 933-6365                    FAX (516) 933-6368
http://www.w2.com/ss.html

Provides information to individuals and professionals through support groups and conferences throughout the U.S., Canada, and abroad.  Membership, U.S., $25.00; Canada, $30.00;  includes bimonthly newsletter, "The Moisture Seekers."

# PUBLICATIONS AND TAPES

After Total-Knee Replacement
Media Services
Sacred Heart Medical Center
PO Box 2555
Spokane, WA 99220-2555
(509) 458-5236                    FAX (509) 626-4475

In this videotape, designed to be viewed prior to surgery, a physical therapist provides instruction in exercises, use of crutches and a walker, and use of the continuous passive motion machine. Includes interviews with individuals who have had knee replacement surgery. 15 minutes. Available in English and Spanish. Purchase, $195.00; rental, $45.00 (may be applied toward purchase); plus $5.00 shipping and handling. Companion booklet, "Home Care Program: Total-Knee Surgery," $1.00. Available in English and Spanish.

Arthritis and Everyday Living
Therapy Skill Builders
555 Academic Court
San Antonio, TX 78204-2498
(800) 228-0752              (800) 723-1318 (TT)              FAX (800) 232-1223
e-mail: customer_service@hbtpc.com

This instructional videotape demonstrates techniques for everyday household activities and shows assistive devices. 30 minutes. Viewer's guide included. $65.00 plus 5% and actual shipping charges.

Arthritis and Pregnancy
Arthritis Foundation
1314 Spring Street, NW
Atlanta, GA 30309
(800) 283-7800              (404) 872-7100              FAX (404) 872-0457
http://www@arthritis.org

This booklet provides information for women with rheumatoid arthritis as well as other forms of arthritis. Discusses how pregnancy affects rheumatoid arthritis and vice versa. Includes a self-test for strength and endurance and suggestions for saving energy and protecting joints when caring for a baby. Free

Arthritis: A Take Care of Yourself Health Guide
by James F. Fries
Addison-Wesley-Longman Publishing Company
1 Jacob Way
Reading, MA 01867
(800) 447-2226              (617) 944-3700

This book describes the major forms of arthritis and methods of managing the condition through exercise, medication, or surgery; describes diagnostic tests; and suggests problem solving techniques for pain, mobility, sexual function, and employment. $14.00

Arthritis, Rheumatic Diseases, and Related Disorders
National Arthritis and Musculoskeletal and Skin Diseases Information Clearinghouse
1 AMS Circle
Bethesda, MD 20892-3675
(301) 495-4484                    (301) 565-2966 (TT)              FAX (301) 587-4352

This 1993 Special Report provides highlights of the research activities sponsored by the National Institutes of Health, including research on rheumatoid arthritis.  Free

Aspirin and Other NSAIDS
Arthritis Foundation
1314 Spring Street, NW
Atlanta, GA 30309
(800) 283-7800                     (404) 872-7100                 FAX (404) 872-0457
http://www@arthritis.org

Using a question and answer format, this booklet discusses NSAIDs and possible side effects.  Free

Coping with Osteoarthritis
by Robert H. Phillips
Avery Publishing Group
120 Old Broadway
Garden City Park, NY 11040
(800) 548-5757                     (516) 741-2155                 FAX (516) 742-1892

Written by a psychologist, this book provides information for individuals and their families on coping with the condition and improving quality of life.  $9.95 plus $3.00 shipping and handling.

Coping with Rheumatoid Arthritis
by Robert H. Phillips
Avery Publishing Group
120 Old Broadway
Garden City Park, NY 11040
(800) 548-5757                     (516) 741-2155                 FAX (516) 742-1892

Written by a psychologist, this book discusses strategies for improving the quality of life; advice for dealing with the emotional aspects of this chronic condition; suggestions for activities and lifestyle changes; and information for family members.  $9.95 plus $3.00 shipping and handling.

Feeling Good With Arthritis
Info Vision
13425 A Street
Omaha, NE 68144
(800) 237-1808                     FAX (402) 330-9544

This videotape discusses the importance of exercise, medical treatment, diet, and attitude.  Individuals with rheumatoid arthritis and osteoarthritis describe their experiences.  60 minutes.  $25.00 plus $5.00 shipping and handling.

Guide to Independent Living for People with Arthritis
Arthritis Foundation
1314 Spring Street, NW
Atlanta, GA 30309
(800) 283-7800                    (404) 872-7100                    FAX (404) 872-0457
http://www@arthritis.org

This book contains photographs of hundreds of adaptive aids that can help individuals with arthritis live independently, with reduced pain. Product descriptions, hints for use, and names and addresses of manufacturers are provided. $10.00

Health, Life and Disability Insurance for People with Arthritis
Arthritis Foundation
1314 Spring Street, NW
Atlanta, GA 30309
(800) 283-7800                    (404) 872-7100                    FAX (404) 872-0457
http://www@arthritis.org

This booklet describes health, life, and disability insurance available through private companies and government programs. Provides checklists to use in buying insurance. Free

Hip Replacement Therapy
Therapy Skill Builders
555 Academic Court
San Antonio, TX 78204-2498
(800) 228-0752                    (800) 723-1318 (TT)                FAX (800) 232-1223
e-mail: customer_service@hbtpc.com

This videotape demonstrates exercise treatment after total hip replacement. 21 minutes. $99.00 plus 5% and actual shipping charges.

Living and Loving: Information About Sex
Arthritis Foundation
1314 Spring Street, NW
Atlanta, GA 30309
(800) 283-7800                    (404) 872-7100                    FAX (404) 872-0457
http://www@arthritis.org

This booklet discusses the effects that medication, physical problems, and emotional responses may have on sexuality in individuals with rheumatic diseases, including rheumatoid arthritis, and their partners. Makes suggestions for improving sexual relations. Free

Living with Arthritis
Resources for Rehabilitation
33 Bedford Street, Suite 19A
Lexington, MA 02173
(617) 862-6455                    FAX (617) 861-7517

One title in a series of large print publications designed for distribution by professionals to people with disabilities. Includes information on how to obtain services, organizations that serve people with arthritis, publications, and aids that help people with arthritis. Minimum purchase, 25 copies. $1.50 per copy plus shipping and handling. Discounts available for purchases of 100 or more copies. (See order form on last page of this book.)

<u>Living with Rheumatoid Arthritis</u>
by Tammi L. Shlotzhauer and James L. McGuire
Johns Hopkins University Press
2715 North Charles Street
Baltimore, MD 21218
(800) 537-5487            FAX (410) 516-6998

Written by two rheumatologists, this book covers the physical aspects of rheumatoid arthritis and medical and surgical treatment, describes coping techniques, suggests exercises, and provides information about everyday activities. $15.95 plus $3.00 shipping and handling.

<u>Managing Your Activities</u>
<u>Managing Your Fatigue</u>
<u>Managing Your Health Care</u>
<u>Managing Your Pain</u>
<u>Managing Your Stress</u>
Arthritis Foundation
1314 Spring Street, NW
Atlanta, GA 30309
(800) 283-7800          (404) 872-7100          FAX (404) 872-0457
http://www@arthritis.org

This series of brochures describes self-management techniques for coping with arthritis. "Managing Your Activities" suggests methods that will enable women to reduce stress on joints affected by arthritis and provides tips for self-help techniques and assistive devices. "Managing Your Fatigue" discusses fatigue, a common symptom in individuals with rheumatic disease. A "Fatigue Care Chart" enables women to identify causes of fatigue and suggests possible solutions. "Managing Your Health Care" describes the roles various health care professionals play in treating individuals with rheumatic diseases. Provides guidelines for making the most of office visits and a list of questions to ask physicians. "Managing Your Pain" discusses pain management strategies such as medication, exercise, assistive devices, heat and cold treatments, massage, and relaxation techniques. "Managing Your Stress" describes how stress can lead to physical and emotional reactions and discusses stress management techniques such as deep breathing, progressive relaxation, guided imagery, and visualization. All are free.

<u>Mother-to-Be: A Guide to Pregnancy and Birth For Women with Disabilities</u>
by Judith Rogers and Molleen Matsumura
Demos Vermande
386 Park Avenue South, Suite 201
New York, NY 10016
(800) 532-8663          (212) 683-0072          FAX (212) 683-0118

This book describes the pregnancy and childbirth experiences of 36 women with a wide variety of disabilities including rheumatoid arthritis. Suggests practical solutions for the special concerns of individuals with disabilities during pregnancy and those of their partners, families, and health care providers. Includes a list of resources, glossary, and bibliography. $24.95 plus $4.00 shipping and handling.

Osteoarthritis
Arthritis Foundation
1314 Spring Street, NW
Atlanta, GA 30309
(800) 283-7800                      (404) 872-7100                      FAX (404) 872-0457
http://www@arthritis.org

This booklet describes the causes, diagnosis, and treatment of osteoarthritis. Includes "joint saver" tips for independent living with reduced pain. Available in English and Spanish. Free

Osteoarthritis
National Arthritis and Musculoskeletal and Skin Diseases Information Clearinghouse
1 AMS Circle
Bethesda, MD 20892
(301) 495-4484                      (301) 565-2966 (TT)                      FAX (301) 587-4352

This information packet contains medical articles, patient information, fact sheets, and a glossary. Also lists Multi-Purpose Arthritis Centers where research is conducted. Free

Osteoarthritis and Rheumatoid Arthritis
Films for the Humanities & Sciences
PO Box 2053
Princeton, NJ 08543-2053
(800) 257-5126                      FAX (609) 275-3767

This videotape describes the differences between these two conditions as well as medical and surgical treatments. 19 minutes. Purchase, $149.00; rental, $75.00; plus $5.75 shipping and handling.

Pain-Free Arthritis
S & J Books
PO Box 276092
Palmetto Park Station
Boca Raton, FL 33427-6092
(561) 368-5726

This videotape and book demonstrate 35 exercises to be done in a swimming pool. Book, $23.85; videotape, $99.00.

People With Arthritis Can Exercise (PACE)
Pool Exercise Program (PEP)
Arthritis Foundation
1314 Spring Street, NW
Atlanta, GA 30309
(800) 283-7800                    (404) 872-7100                    FAX (404) 872-0457
http://www@arthritis.org

These videotapes present different levels and types of exercise programs. "PACE Level 1" is a gentle exercise program for individuals with significant joint disease; $18.50. "PACE Level 2" is a moderate exercise program designed to increase endurance for individuals with mild arthritis; $19.50. PEP is an aquatic exercise program; $19.50. Add $4.00 shipping and handling.

Rebuilding Arthritic Hands
Films for the Humanities & Sciences
PO Box 2053
Princeton, NJ 08543-2053
(800) 257-5126                    FAX (609) 275-3767

This videotape describes surgical and nonsurgical treatment for arthritis in the hand. 21 minutes. $89.95 plus $5.75 shipping and handling.

Rheumatoid Arthritis
Arthritis Foundation
1314 Spring Street, NW
Atlanta, GA 30309
(800) 283-7800                    (404) 872-7100                    FAX (404) 872-0457
http://www@arthritis.org

This booklet describes rheumatoid arthritis and explains how it differs from other forms of arthritis. Discusses diagnostic tests and treatment with medications, rest, exercise, and surgery. Available in English and Spanish. Free

Sjogren's Syndrome
Arthritis Foundation
1314 Spring Street, NW
Atlanta, GA  30309
(800) 283-7800                    (404) 872-7100                    FAX (404) 872-0457
http://www@arthritis.org

This booklet explains the causes, symptoms, diagnosis, and treatment for this related condition. Free

The Sjogren's Syndrome Handbook
Sjogren's Syndrome Foundation
333 North Broadway
Jericho, NY 11753
(800) 475-6473                    (516) 933-6365                    FAX (516) 933-6368
http://www.w2.com/ss.html

This book provides practical suggestions for living more comfortably with this chronic condition. Members, $19.95; nonmembers, $29.95; plus $2.50 shipping and handling; shipping to Canada, $7.00.

Total-Hip Replacement: Stride to Recovery
Media Services
Sacred Heart Medical Center
PO Box 2555
Spokane, WA 99220-2555
(509) 458-5236                    FAX (509) 626-4475

In this videotape, two individuals describe their hospitalization; share tips on home adaptations; and discuss safety precautions. 12 minutes. Available in English and Spanish. Purchase, $195.00; rental, $45.00 (may be applied toward purchase); plus $5.00 shipping and handling. Companion booklet, "Your New Total Hip," $2.00. Available in English and Spanish.

Understanding Osteoarthritis  19 minutes
Understanding Rheumatoid Arthritis  22 minutes
by James Brodie
Fanlight Productions
47 Halifax Street
Boston, MA 02130
(800) 937-4113                    (617) 542-0980                    FAX (617) 542-8838
e-mail: fanlight@tiac.net         http://www.fanlight.com

In these videotapes, each condition is described as well as its treatment, pain relief, and lifestyle changes. Interviews with people living with arthritis are included. Purchase, $99.00; rental, $50.00; plus $9.00 per title shipping and handling.

# Chapter 5

## *DIABETES*

Diabetes mellitus is a term that applies to a variety of disorders related to the production or utilization of insulin, a substance that is necessary to metabolize the glucose (sugar) that the body needs for energy. As a result of diabetes, the body is unable to maintain normal glucose levels. *Hypoglycemia* is a condition where the level of glucose is too low. It occurs when the individual does not eat soon enough or eats too little, uses too much insulin, or engages in overactivity. Hypoglycemia may lead to an insulin reaction; symptoms may include feeling shaky or sweaty, headache, hunger, irritability, and dizziness. Insulin shock sometimes occurs if an insulin reaction is not treated quickly; in these cases individuals may lose consciousness. *Hyperglycemia* is a condition where the level of glucose in the blood is too high. Symptoms include extreme thirst, a dry mouth, excessive urination, blurred vision, and lethargy. Sometimes when an individual who has had an insulin reaction takes food high in sugar to replace glucose in the body, too much glucose is released, resulting in high blood glucose levels (hyperglycemia). The combination of too much sugar without enough insulin to use it properly may gradually lead to diabetic coma if warning signs are not monitored; diabetic coma usually occurs only in individuals with insulin-dependent diabetes.

About 6.5 million Americans, or 2.6% of the population, have been diagnosed with diabetes. Diabetes is an age related disease, with those age 65 or over having the highest rates; nearly three million elders have been diagnosed with diabetes. However, half the people who have diabetes are not aware of it (Centers for Disease Control: 1993). In every age range, proportionately more women have diabetes than men, with 27.0 women per thousand known to have diabetes compared to 22.2 men per thousand overall (National Center for Health Statistics: 1987a). African-American females had the highest prevalence rate of diabetes during the years 1980 to 1990 followed by African-American males. The prevalence rates of diabetes for white females surpassed the rates for white males during the same period (Centers for Disease Control: 1993). Women who have diabetes are at risk during pregnancy, as are their fetuses, and must take special precautions. In addition, some women develop diabetes during pregnancy (gestational diabetes mellitus) and are at risk for the disease following pregnancy as well (see "Types of Diabetes," "Sexual Functioning," and "Family Planning, Pregnancy, and Childrearing" sections below).

Diabetes was the third most frequent primary diagnosis for individuals who visited outpatient departments in non-federal hospitals in 1994 (Lipkind: 1996). More than half (57.5%) of the 13.2 million patient visits to physicians in 1989 that had a primary diagnosis of diabetes were made by women (Schappert: 1992). Diabetes and its complications are responsible for many hospital stays and have a large economic impact on society. A recent study indicated that individuals with diabetes spent more than four times as much in 1992 on health care costs as individuals without diabetes (Rubin et al.: 1994).

Currently, there is no cure for diabetes; however, there are means to control the disease and to decrease the risk of the numerous associated complications. Early diagnosis and intervention are crucial steps in maintaining proper control of diabetes.

Transplantations of the pancreas (the gland responsible for secreting insulin), although no longer considered experimental, are performed only in a select group of patients. Currently, transplantations are performed on patients who have end-stage renal disease, have had or plan to have a kidney transplant as well, have serious clinical difficulty with insulin injections, and do not present an excessive risk for this type of surgery (American Diabetes Association: 1996a). When successful, pancreas transplantation results in the elimination of insulin injections. Rejection of transplanted tissue and the need for large amounts of immunosuppressive drugs are important factors that have prevented this type of transplantation from becoming standard procedure. Because people with diabetes are especially prone to infection, transplantation involves more risks for this population than for other individuals. Research to improve the management of diabetes through innovative administration of insulin and drugs that improve the body's use of insulin is ongoing. Transplantation of islet cells in the pancreas that are responsible for insulin production is also under investigation.

## *TYPES OF DIABETES*

The two major types of diabetes mellitus are referred to as Type I and Type II. In *Type I*, the pancreas does not produce insulin. Individuals with Type I diabetes must take regular injections of insulin. For this reason, Type I is also referred to as Insulin-Dependent Diabetes Mellitus (IDDM). This variant of the disease was formerly called juvenile-onset diabetes, because it is usually diagnosed at a young age. Symptoms of Type I diabetes include extreme thirst, weight loss despite increased appetite, weakness and fatigue, and blurred vision.

In the United States there are an estimated 300,000 to 500,000 individuals with insulin-dependent diabetes mellitus (IDDM) (National Institute of Diabetes and Digestive and Kidney Diseases: 1990). In addition to daily insulin injections, individuals with IDDM must carefully watch their diet and coordinate meals with insulin doses to maintain a balanced glucose level. Insulin may be injected by syringe or by "jet injectors" that do not use actual needles. Some individuals, especially those who are on erratic schedules that prevent them from eating on a regular schedule, use insulin pumps that automatically provide insulin throughout the day. The use of insulin pumps often results in improved control of blood glucose levels over other methods. Prior to eating, pump users determine the amount of insulin they need and program the pump to release that amount.

In *Type II* diabetes, the body produces some insulin but does not produce enough or does not utilize it properly. Because Type II diabetes usually does not require insulin injections, it is also referred to as noninsulin-dependent diabetes mellitus (NIDDM). This type of the disease is often called adult-onset or maturity-onset diabetes, because it is most frequently diagnosed after age forty. It is estimated that over 90% of the cases of diabetes in the United States are Type II (National Center for Health Statistics: 1987b).

Although the causes of Type II diabetes are not known, obesity (80 to 90% of all individuals with Type II diabetes are obese) and a family history of diabetes are predisposing factors. Symptoms of noninsulin-dependent diabetes include fatigue, frequent urination, excessive thirst, and vaginal infections in women. Individuals who have these symptoms should make an appointment for a physical examination. However, diabetes is sometimes present when no symptoms are evident (Williams: 1983). Tests for glucose in urine or a blood glucose test conducted during a routine physical examination are often the first indications of diabetes.

In many cases, noninsulin-dependent diabetes can be controlled through both diet and exercise. For obese individuals who have diabetes, a change in diet and reduction of caloric intake may make a dramatic difference in blood glucose levels. Research suggests that individuals with Type II diabetes may lower their blood glucose and insulin levels throughout the day by increasing the frequency and decreasing the size of their meals. This strategy slows the rate of carbohydrate absorption. A possible disadvantage is that obese individuals who use this dietary plan may have a tendency to gain weight (Jenkins: 1995).

Diet and exercise for people with either type of diabetes should be planned with a physician's advice to ensure that all medical conditions are taken into account. The goals of dietary restrictions are to reduce total body weight and to minimize the intake of glucose. The American Diabetes Association has produced many publications about diet for people with diabetes, including "Exchange

Lists" (developed jointly with the American Dietetic Association), which list foods with similar caloric and nutrient contents (see "PUBLICATIONS AND TAPES" section below).

Exercise helps the body to utilize the glucose and thus is an important part of the plan to control diabetes. In some individuals with Type II diabetes, the muscle cells that are receptors for glucose do not work efficiently; exercise enables muscle cells to use the glucose efficiently without requiring more insulin (Cantu: 1982). Exercise also reduces fat, which is known to reduce the body's sensitivity to insulin. After consulting with a physician, even individuals who have been sedentary can begin a gradual exercise program by starting to take brief daily walks. A regular exercise regimen has been shown to be useful in reducing the required levels of daily insulin injections.

When diet and exercise are insufficient to control Type II diabetes, oral medications are prescribed. Sulfonylureas are a type of medication that causes the pancreas to produce increased amounts of insulin. Side effects of this type of medication include hypoglycemia and hyperinsulinemia, a condition in which too much insulin is in the bloodstream. Hyperinsulinemia is a risk factor for vascular disease and heart attack. In addition, sulfonylureas often fail to work after a number of years, as the pancreas can no longer produce sufficient insulin. When this occurs, individuals must begin injecting insulin. Several drugs that use different mechanisms to control diabetes are currently being tested.

One drug that has been available throughout much of the world since the late 1950's, metformin (Glucophage), has recently been approved for use in the United States. Although it is not clear exactly how metformin works, it is effective in lowering blood glucose levels and has no serious side effects, unless the individual has kidney disease at the outset. Another drug recently approved by the Food and Drug Administration is acarbose, a carbohydrase inhibitor. Carbohydrases are the enzymes that break down carbohydrates and turn them into glucose. The side effects of acarbose are bloating, gas, and diarrhea, which may subside after six months of taking the drug (American Diabetes Association: 1995).

Although testing urine for sugar was previously used to monitor glucose levels, this method is not as accurate as testing the blood directly. People with both types of diabetes use home blood glucose monitoring equipment to measure glucose levels; this involves putting a drop of blood from a fingertip on a specially treated strip designed to react to the glucose. The color of the strip indicates the level of glucose that is present. A digital display or speech output indicates the blood glucose level, and some monitors record the date and time of the reading. Illness, even a simple cold, can affect how the body uses insulin; glucose monitoring is even more important at these times. Log booklets enable individuals to keep a record of their blood glucose levels and to analyze their diets and schedules to determine what causes them to have varying levels of blood glucose. Home blood glucose monitors are inexpensive and are quite compact, making them suitable for travel and to take to work or school.

Diabetes adds a financial burden that is often not covered by medical insurance. Although the initial cost of a blood glucose monitor is relatively low, the cost of the strips that are used to test the blood, supplies to inject insulin, and special foods increase a woman's expenditures substantially. The financial burden of managing diabetes often prevents women with low to moderate income from taking proper care of themselves. Some women are forced to sacrifice normal expenditures in order to meet these expenses.

Both types of diabetes have the same potential long term health effects. It is essential that everyone with diabetes be aware of the proper management of their disease and all of the potential complications. Complications of diabetes include greater risks of heart disease, stroke, infections, and nephropathy (kidney disease); circulatory problems that can be especially problematic for legs and feet (resulting in amputation in extreme cases); neuropathy or nerve disease which causes tingling, numbness, double vision, pain, or dizziness; and vision problems. Good control of blood glucose levels can help to prevent these long term complications.

Among the leading vision problems caused by diabetes is diabetic retinopathy. Visual impairment occurs when the small blood vessels in the retina are damaged and fail to nourish the retina adequately. One consequence of this process is bleeding inside the eye. If detected early, diabetic retinopathy can sometimes be treated successfully by laser therapy. In other cases, complex surgical procedures are performed in the attempt to restore useful vision. To manage their diabetes, many people with visual impairments use a wide range of adapted equipment, such as glucometers, scales, and thermometers with speech output; syringe magnifiers; special insulin gauges; and special syringes that automatically measure insulin doses.

The Diabetes Control and Complications Trial (1993) recently reported the results of a study which monitored 1,441 individuals with Type I diabetes who were assigned to receive either conventional therapy (one or two injections of insulin daily) or intensive therapy (three or more injections of insulin daily). Results indicate that the intensive therapy group had significantly lower incidence of retinopathy, nephropathy, and neuropathy. The chief adverse effect of intensive therapy was increased episodes of severe hypoglycemia. Although the effects of intensive therapy have not been tested on people with Type II diabetes, many practitioners believe that the results are also applicable to this type of diabetes.

Women with diabetes may notice a dramatic increase in blood glucose two to five days before menstruation begins. During the week before menstruation begins, the levels of estrogen and progesterone are at their highest levels; since these two hormones exert an anti-insulin effect, it takes more than the usual amount of insulin to control blood glucose. Once menstruation begins and the levels of these hormones drop, blood glucose levels also drop. Women must experiment with insulin dosages to determine the adjustments that are necessary during the various phases of the menstrual cycle (Jovanovic et al.: 1987).

Women with diabetes are especially susceptible to vaginal infections. When blood glucose is high, yeast infections are more likely. Vaginal infections are a common symptom of undiagnosed diabetes. Uncontrolled diabetes may also result in missed menstrual periods.

Menopause results in a decreased need for insulin due to decreased levels of estrogen and progesterone and may result in low blood glucose levels. Because women with Type I diabetes have usually had the disease for 20 years or more when they reach menopause, they are likely to have developed neuropathy and not to be sensitive to the symptoms of hypoglycemia (Jovanovic et al.: 1987).

*Gestational diabetes mellitus* (GDM) occurs in approximately three percent of all pregnancies in the United States, usually in the third trimester of pregnancy (Engelau et al.: 1995). Recent efforts to screen all pregnant women for gestational diabetes between the 24th and 28th week of pregnancy have resulted in a dramatic decrease in the perinatal* mortality rate among pregnant women with this form of diabetes. Screening for gestational diabetes consists of an oral glucose tolerance test (OGTT), in which the mother ingests glucose and has her blood glucose tested one hour afterward. If the result is abnormal (140mg/dl or higher), she must return for a fasting oral glucose tolerance test and have her blood glucose tested after an overnight fast of at least eight hours and at one, two, and three hours after ingesting the glucose. Insulin does not cross the placenta, but glucose does, causing the baby's pancreas to produce extra insulin (American Diabetes Association: 1996b). Macrosomia, a condition in which the baby's weight is abnormally high and a possible complication of gestational diabetes, may cause injury to the baby if the delivery is difficult; it may also result in obesity in childhood.

---

*shortly before and after birth, usually defined as the 29th week of gestation until 4 weeks after birth

Treatment for gestational diabetes usually consists of dietary therapy and self-monitoring of blood glucose. If the woman is still hyperglycemic, she may be treated with insulin (Centers for Disease Control: 1991). In some instances when the woman has difficulty controlling blood glucose, she may be hospitalized.

Half or more of all women who develop gestational diabetes will develop diabetes at some point later in life. Therefore, women with gestational diabetes should be screened for diabetes at six to eight weeks after delivery and have annual screenings thereafter. Women with gestational diabetes should be educated about the symptoms of diabetes and should consult a physician if the symptoms appear.

## SEXUAL FUNCTIONING

It has been suggested that the sexual functioning of women with diabetes may be affected in several ways, including reduced sexual libido and ability to achieve orgasm. The relatively few studies that have been carried out on this subject have resulted in contradictory findings. Some studies have found that women with diabetes do have reduced libido and are less likely to achieve orgasm, while other studies find no significant differences between women with diabetes and those who do not have diabetes (Schreiner-Engel: 1983; Wilson Young and Barthalow Koch: 1989). Methodological differences among the studies and the use of self-reports limit the validity of these studies.

Depression upon the diagnosis of the disease may interfere with sexual desire. The woman's partner may also be depressed and, without adequate information about the disease, may avoid sexual relations. Diabetes that is out of control may result in vaginal infections and lack of vaginal lubrication, causing painful intercourse. Neuropathy, which usually occurs only after a woman has had diabetes for many years, may affect the genitals and cause lack of sensation or painful intercourse.

## FAMILY PLANNING, PREGNANCY, AND CHILDREARING

Women with diabetes are able to become pregnant, although historically the rate of complications has been much higher for women with diabetes than for those who do not have diabetes. Congenital malformations of babies born to mothers with overt or established diabetes (diabetes that was not caused by the pregnancy) include those of the central nervous system, skeleton, heart, and kidneys (Centers for Disease Control: 1991). Rates of cesarean delivery, spontaneous abortion, and preterm labor are high, as are risks to the mother's health. Acceptable blood glucose levels for pregnant women are lower than normal, because hyperglycemia is associated with increased morbidity and mortality for both the mother and the fetus. Achieving this tight control often results in episodes of hypoglycemia. Women with diabetes may use most of the methods of birth control that other women use. Birth control pills should be low dosage, and women who have high blood pressure should not use them (Jovanovic et al.: 1987).

Diabetes was present in 4% of all pregnancies in the United States in 1988. Gestational diabetes accounted for most of the cases (88%), noninsulin-dependent diabetes accounted for 8% of the cases, and insulin-dependent diabetes for 4%. Mothers with gestational diabetes and those with noninsulin-dependent diabetes were older than mothers whose pregnancies were not complicated by diabetes. Both age and obesity were associated with the development of gestational diabetes (Engelau et al.: 1995).

Women who have advanced diabetic retinopathy are at risk for exacerbating the disease if they become pregnant. A recent study (Chew et al.: 1995) found that women whose diabetes was poorly controlled and who had retinopathy at conception were more likely to have progression of their retinopathy during pregnancy than women who had no retinopathy or only microaneurysms. The researchers recommended that women with diabetes and retinopathy who are contemplating pregnancy bring their diabetes into tight control prior to conception.

Women with diabetes who have kidney disease or nephropathy who become pregnant may experience an acceleration of the progression of the disease (Purdy et al.: 1996) and are at risk for preeclampsia (Centers for Disease Control: 1991), a condition which occurs in the third trimester of pregnancy or during labor. For these reasons, it is often recommended that women with diabetes who have kidney disease not become pregnant (Jovanovic et al.: 1987). Preeclampsia involves elevation of blood pressure, protein in the urine, abdominal pain, edema (abnormal accumulation of fluids), visual disturbances, and headache. Preeclampsia often requires preterm delivery of the baby. Eclampsia, a condition that occurs in about five percent of the cases of preeclampsia, causes convulsions and coma and may be life threatening (Margolis and Greenwood: 1993). Women with nephropathy who do decide to become pregnant must monitor not only their blood glucose but also their blood pressure, keeping it at 130/85 or lower, according to John Kitzmiller, a physician who specializes in the care of pregnant women with diabetes. Blood pressure may be kept in control through the use of medications, although pregnant women with diabetes may not use all of the blood pressure medications available to the general population, as some of these medications may affect the fetus and glycemic control. Recommended medications are methyldopa, prazosin, or clonidine (American Diabetes Association: 1996c).

Women who plan to become pregnant are advised to seek preconception counseling and care in order to be certain that their blood glucose is maintained at levels that will minimize risks to themselves and their babies. Preconception and perinatal care have proven to be successful in reducing infant morbidity and mortality as well as reducing the number of cesarean section deliveries (Catalano: 1988). Glycemic control affects the formation of organs during the first weeks of pregnancy. Therefore, having blood glucose in control before becoming pregnant and maintaining excellent control is crucial to the health of the baby. Jovanovic (1987) recommends that pregnant women with diabetes test their blood glucose five to ten times daily.

Rosenn and colleagues (1991) compared a group of women who attended a preconception program with those who attended a program early in their pregnancy. Those who attended the program before conceiving achieved better glycemic control and experienced lower rates of spontaneous abortion. These clinicians suggested that the results may have differed for the two groups because it often takes several weeks to attain optimal glycemic control and fetal organs had already begun developing during this period in the pregnant group. Despite the recognized importance of preconceptual planning, many women who have diabetes do not receive this counseling from their physicians. A recent study found that less than half of women who sought care after becoming pregnant had ever received any advice about pregnancy from their physicians (Janz et al.: 1995).

Women with Type I diabetes must adjust their insulin dosage throughout their pregnancy. During the first trimester of pregnancy, diabetes is often unstable; stability in the next trimester is followed by an increased need for insulin at about 24 weeks. The increased need for insulin is due to the production of pregnancy related hormones, such as estrogen and progesterone, which act as insulin antagonists (Steel et al.: 1994).

A recent study (Towner et al.: 1995) of pregnant women with Type II diabetes who had not received preconception counseling found that the rate of congenital anomalies among this group of women was similar to the rate for women with Type I diabetes. Control of blood glucose and the mother's age at onset of diabetes were the only variables that had a significant influence upon congenital anomalies. Type of treatment (dietary regimen, insulin injections, or oral agents) did not result in significantly different rates of anomalies.

Macrosomia, a condition in which babies' birth weight is abnormally high, occurs in approximately a quarter of all babies born to women with diabetes. Macrosomia is associated with protracted labor, skeletal and nerve injuries, perinatal asphyxia, and high rates of hypoglycemia in the infants (Cordero and Landon: 1993). The cause of macrosomia in women with diabetes is not fully understood. Recent studies have revealed little relationship between the mother's glycemic control and macrosomia, although it is known that the fetus's own pancreas produces excess amounts of insulin in the third trimester and causes the growth of the fetus (Schwartz et al.: 1994). Macrosomia may necessitate cesarean delivery. Often these babies become obese in childhood and develop glucose intolerance at an early age.

## *PSYCHOLOGICAL ASPECTS OF DIABETES*

Although shock, fear, and depression are normal reactions to diabetes at first, these emotions may subside once the woman understands how to control the disease. Because diabetes affects so many parts of the body, it also affects many aspects of daily life. In addition to prescribed changes in diet and exercise, women with diabetes must always be aware of the symptoms that indicate hyperglycemia or hypoglycemia. Women who must take daily injections of insulin may have to overcome a fear of needles; talking with others who have experienced this fear and overcome it may prove extremely valuable.

Changes in daily routines are never accepted readily. For women with diabetes, changes in lifestyle and the need to monitor glucose may cause great stress. Social events and travel must be carefully planned to ensure that meals will comply with special diets.

Diabetes has a great effect on family relationships as well. The need to make a change in lifestyle may be upsetting not only to the woman herself, but also to her partner and to her children. Planning diets carefully means extra time devoted to shopping and cooking; exercising also takes time away from other family activities. Involving family members in these activities can channel positive energy into helping the woman with diabetes instead of isolating her from her family. All family members should also learn about blood glucose monitoring and insulin injection as well as recognizing the symptoms of insulin reaction and the necessary measures to counter it.

A common fear of mothers is that they will have an insulin reaction when home alone with their babies or young children. Teaching young children how to recognize signs of an insulin reaction and how to call for emergency help may prove to be lifesaving. Numerous incidents have been reported where small children dialed "911" and saved their mothers' lives.

The diagnosis of diabetes may result in the fear that most food is off limits and that it will be impossible to enjoy eating. Recent policy recommendations from the American Diabetes Association (1994) indicate that the use of simple sugars such as sucrose (table sugar) is not off limits and that they do not cause greater or more rapid rises in blood glucose than other carbohydrates. Scientific evidence suggests that sucrose has a similar effect on blood glucose as bread, rice, and potatoes. It is important to keep in mind the total amount of carbohydrates consumed and that simple sugars must be used in place of other carbohydrates in the diet. With the new food labeling laws mandated by the federal government, this calculation becomes much easier, as the amount of carbohydrates per serving must be indicated on the food label. In order to control the amount of carbohydrates, many foods, including desserts and candies, are sweetened with artificial sweeteners or fruit juices.

A number of food manufacturers cater to the dietary needs of individuals with diabetes, and their products are often available in the dietetic food section of large supermarkets. Health food or natural food stores also carry many products that are amenable to the diet of people with diabetes. Perseverance in tracking down the right foods will allow for an interesting and varied diet; however, the shock and depression that follow the diagnosis of diabetes may limit the individual's emotional endurance. Support from a family member or close friend can help women with diabetes to carry out this endeavor.

Public libraries are a good source for the myriad cookbooks that have been written especially for people with diabetes. Discovering the variety of interesting recipes, including those for dessert and candies, should prove to be a psychological boost for women who fear being restricted to bland meals.

Diligent efforts to control glucose by following the recommended dosages of insulin or diets do not always result in the desired response. Women whose glucose is out of control should learn not to feel guilty; they may need to have their insulin or medication dosage and diet modified by a health care professional.

A common response to adult-onset or Type II diabetes is that "It's just a touch of diabetes." This response can be extremely dangerous when the woman fails to properly monitor and control the disease. Women with diabetes and their family members must discuss the disease and its potential effects so that they understand the importance of the prescribed dietary regimen, exercise, and blood glucose monitoring.

Older women with diabetes may experience other disabling conditions or diseases; the additional diagnosis of diabetes may cause them to have grave concerns about their health and their ability to live independently. Widows and older women who live alone may be especially vulnerable to this response. Their physicians may tell them not to worry about the diabetes, because it takes many years to develop serious complications. This attitude may contribute to the woman's denial of her disease and result in exacerbation of the symptoms of hyperglycemia discussed above.

## PROFESSIONAL SERVICE PROVIDERS

Because diabetes is a systemic disease, it has a wide range of effects. As a result, many types of health care professionals are involved in caring for women with diabetes.

*Family physicians* and *internists* are the physicians in charge of coordinating the various aspects of care for individuals with diabetes. *Diabetologists* (endocrinologists) are physicians who specialize in the treatment of individuals with diabetes. *Obstetricians/gynecologists* care for women who are pregnant and treat conditions affecting women's reproductive organs; diabetes makes women susceptible to vaginal infections and puts them at high risk during pregnancy. Obstetricians should work with internists or diabetologists, neonatologists, and diabetes educators to ensure the health of both the mother and the fetus. Some women get their prenatal care from specialists in high risk pregnancies. *Nephrologists* are physicians who treat people with kidney disease, which is a common complication of diabetes. *Ophthalmologists* are physicians who specialize in diseases of the eye. If diabetic retinopathy is detected, individuals are often referred to subspecialists called retina and vitreous specialists.

*Certified diabetes educators* (CDE) are health care professionals certified by the American Association of Diabetes Educators to teach individuals with diabetes how to effectively manage their disease. Certified diabetes educators may be physicians or nurses. Many are dietitians or nutritionists who help people with diabetes plan a diet to control their blood glucose levels.

*Psychologists*, *social workers*, and other counselors help people with diabetes and their family members adjust to the regimen prescribed to control the diabetes.

## WHERE TO FIND SERVICES

In some areas, special treatment centers for diabetes and dialysis centers for people with kidney disease are available. Diabetes treatment centers often have special divisions for the monitoring and care of pregnant women with diabetes. The special physicians listed above practice in hospitals or have private practices. Affiliates of the American Diabetes Association (ADA) exist in every state. These affiliates may provide publications, educational programs, and referrals to local resources. The national office (described in the "ORGANIZATIONS" section below) can provide the address and phone number of local affiliates. The ADA also has information about local support groups. Understanding that others with diabetes continue to live fulfilling lives can be an extremely important benefit of attending support groups. People with diabetes who have vision problems may obtain services from public or private rehabilitation agencies serving individuals who are visually impaired or blind.

## *ASSISTIVE DEVICES*

Individuals with insulin-dependent diabetes use a variety of devices to administer their insulin, such as syringes; insulin pens which combine the insulin dose and injector; needle-free jet injectors; and insulin pumps, which automatically deliver insulin slowly throughout the day and night through a plastic tube attached to a needle. Equipment to measure blood glucose is necessary for both Type I and Type II forms of diabetes. Some health insurance policies will pay some of the costs for glucose monitors and test strips. It is wise to check with the insurance carrier before purchasing such equipment.

Supplies and equipment to help individuals with diabetes to monitor and manage their disease are usually available at pharmacies or medical supply stores. Mail order catalogues also sell these supplies.

## *HOW TO RECOGNIZE AN INSULIN REACTION AND GIVE FIRST AID*

Individuals experiencing an insulin reaction may feel shaky or dizzy, sweat profusely, complain of a headache, or act irritable. Family members of the woman with diabetes, including her children, should learn the signs of insulin reaction. Suggestions for giving first aid to individuals who have had an insulin reaction are:

- Give the individual some food, such as orange juice, milk, or even sugar itself, to replace the low blood sugar level. Many individuals with diabetes carry sugar packets, glucose tablets, or candy with them for use in emergencies.
- If the individual is unconscious, rub honey or another sugary substance into the mouth, between the teeth and cheek.

Frequent insulin reactions should be reported to the physician. It is recommended that individuals with diabetes wear a medical identification bracelet so that emergency care personnel will know that they have diabetes.

References

American Diabetes Association
1996a "Pancreas Transplantation for Patients with Diabetes Mellitus" Diabetes Care 19(January):Supplement 1:S39
1996b "Why Worry about Gestational Diabetes?" Diabetes Forecast 49(March):3:46-47
1996c "Pregnancy and Beyond" Diabetes Forecast 49(September):9:31-32
1995 "Surge Protector" Diabetes Forecast 48(May)5:23-24

1994   "Nutrition Recommendations and Principles for People with Diabetes Mellitus" <u>Diabetes Care</u> 17(May)5:519-522

Cantu, Robert C.

1982   <u>Diabetes and Exercise</u>  New York, NY: E.P. Dutton

Catalano, Patrick M.

1988   "Diabetic Pregnancy: Is It Time to Enjoy the Fruits of Our Labor?"   <u>Diabetes Care</u> 11(November):292-293

Centers for Disease Control

1993   <u>Diabetes Surveillance, 1993</u> Atlanta, GA: Public Health Service

1991   <u>The Prevention and Treatment of Complications of Diabetes</u> Atlanta, GA: Public Health Service

Chew, Emily et al.

1995   "Metabolic Control and Progression of Retinopathy" <u>Diabetes Care</u> 18(May):5:631-637

Cordero, Leandro and Mark B. Landon

1993   "Infant of the Diabetic Mother" <u>Clinics in Perinatology</u> 20(September)3:635-648

Diabetes Control and Complications Trial Research Group

1993   "The Effect of Intensive Treatment of Diabetes on the Development and Progression of Long-Term Complications in Insulin-Dependent Diabetes Mellitus"   <u>New England Journal of Medicine</u>  329(September 30):14:977-986

Engelau, Michael et al.

1995   "The Epidemiology of Diabetes and Pregnancy in the U.S., 1988" <u>Diabetes Care</u> 18(July):7:1029-1033

Janz, Nancy K. et al.

1995   "Diabetes and Pregnancy" <u>Diabetes Care</u> 18(February)2:157-165

Jenkins, David J. A.

1995   "Nutritional Principles and Diabetes" <u>Diabetes Care</u> 18(November)11:1491-1498

Jovanovic, Lois, June Biermann, and Barbara Toohey

1987   <u>The Diabetic Woman</u> Los Angeles, CA: Jeremy P. Tarcher

Lipkind, Karen L.

1996   "National Hospital Ambulatory Medical Care Survey: 1994 Outpatient Department Summary" <u>Advance Data from Vital and Health Statistics</u>, No. 276, Hyattsville, MD: National Center for Health Statistics, June 11

Margolis, Alan J. and Sadja Greenwood

1993   "Gynecology and Obstetrics"  pp. 560-613 in Lawrence M. Tierney, Jr. et al. (eds.) <u>Current Medical Diagnosis and Treatment</u> Englewood Cliffs, NJ: Appleton and Lange

National Center for Health Statistics

1987a "Prevalence of Known Diabetes among Black Americans" <u>Advance Data from Vital and Health Statistics</u>, No. 130, DHHS Pub. No. (PHS) 87-1250.  Public Health Service, Hyattsville, MD July 31, 1987

1987b "Health Practices and Perceptions of U.S. Adults with Noninsulin-Dependent Diabetes.  Data from the 1985 National Health Interview Survey of Health Promotion and Disease Prevention" <u>Advance Data from Vital and Health Statistics</u>, No. 141, DHHS Pub. No. (PHS) 87-1250. Public Health Service, Hyattsville, MD  September 23, 1987

National Institute of Diabetes and Digestive and Kidney Diseases

1990   <u>Insulin-Dependent Diabetes</u>  Bethesda, MD: National Diabetes Information Clearinghouse

Purdy, Lisa P. et al.

1996   "Effect of Pregnancy on Renal Function in Patients with Moderate-to-Severe Diabetic Renal Insufficiency" <u>Diabetes Care</u> 19(October):10:1067-1074

Rosenn, Barak et al.

1991 "Pre-Conception Management of Insulin-Dependent Diabetes: Improvement of Pregnancy Outcome" Obstetrics and Gynecology 77(June):6:846-849

Rubin, Robert J., William M. Altman, and Daniel N. Mendelson

1994 "Health Care Expenditures for People with Diabetes Mellitus, 1992" Journal of Clinical Endocrinology and Metabolism 78:4:809A-809F

Schappert, Susan M.

1992 "Office Visits for Diabetes Mellitus: United States, 1989" Advance Data from Vital and Health Statistics No. 211, DHHS Pub. No. (PHS) 92-1250. Hyattsville, MD: Public Health Service March 24, 1992

Schreiner-Engel, Patricia

1983 "Diabetes Mellitus and Female Sexuality" Sexuality and Disability 6(Summer):2:83-92

Schwartz, Robert et al.

1994 "Hyperinsulinemia and Macrosomia in the Fetus of the Diabetic Mother" Diabetes Care 17(July):7:640-649

Steel, Judith M. et al.

1994 "Insulin Requirements During Pregnancy in Women with Type I Diabetes" Obstetrics and Gynecology 83(February):2:253-258

Towner, Dena et al.

1995 "Congenital Malformations in Pregnancies Complicated by NIDDM" Diabetes Care 18(November):1:1446-1451

Williams, T. Franklin

1983 "Diabetes Mellitus in Older People" pp. 411-415 in William Reichel (ed.) Clinical Aspects of Aging Baltimore, MD: Williams and Wilkins

Wilson Young, Elaine and Patricia Barthalow Koch

1989 "Research Comparing the Dyadic Adjustment and Sexual Functioning Concerns of Diabetic and Nondiabetic Women" Health Care for Women International 10:377-394

# *ORGANIZATIONS*

American Amputee Foundation
PO Box 250218
Little Rock, AR 72225
(501) 666-2523

A national information clearinghouse and referral center. Provides technical assistance in starting self-help groups and sponsors self-help groups across the country. Membership, $25.00, includes newsletter and "AAF National Resource Directory."

American Association of Diabetes Educators (AADE)
444 North Michigan Avenue, Suite 1240
Chicago, IL 60611
(800) 338-3633                    (312) 644-2233                    FAX (312) 644-4411

Membership organization for health care professionals who work with people with diabetes. Holds annual meeting. Membership, $75.00, includes a bimonthly journal, "The Diabetes Educator." Journal only, U.S., $45.00; foreign, $52.00.

American Association of Kidney Patients (AAKP)
100 South Ashley Drive, Suite 280
Tampa, FL 33606
(800) 749-2257                    (813) 223-7099                    FAX (813) 223-0001

Advocates on behalf of patients with kidney disease; sponsors local patient and family support groups; holds conferences and seminars. Membership, patient/family, $15.00; professional, $30.00; includes newsletter, "AAKP Bulletin" and a magazine, "Renal Life."

American Diabetes Association (ADA)
1660 Duke Street
Alexandria, VA  22314
(800) 232-3472                    In the Washington, DC, (703) 549-1500
FAX (703) 836-7439               http://www.diabetes.org

National membership organization with local affiliates. Publications for both professionals and consumers, including cookbooks and guides for the management of diabetes (see "PUBLICATIONS AND TAPES" section below). Consumer membership, U.S., $24.00; Canada, $41.73; Mexico, $39.00; foreign, $49.00; includes a 10% discount on publications, a subscription to "Diabetes Forecast" (also available on disc from the National Library Service) which includes articles and information about special diabetes products and vendors, and membership in a local affiliate. Professional membership levels vary. Many local affiliates offer their own publications, sponsor support groups, and conduct professional training programs. The World Wide Web site includes featured articles from "Diabetes Forecast" and the medical journal "Diabetes Care."

American Kidney Fund
6110 Executive Boulevard, Suite 1010
Rockville, MD 20852
(800) 638-8299                    (301) 881-3052                    FAX (301) 881-0898

Provides public and professional education and financial aid to individuals who have chronic kidney problems.


Amputee Coalition of America (ACA)
6300 River Road, Suite 727
Rosemont, IL 60018-4226
(708) 698-1633

Provides education and support services to individuals with amputations through a network of peer support groups, educational programs for health professionals, and a database of resources. Membership, individuals, $15.00; professionals, $50.00; amputee support groups, $25.00; includes newsletter, "ACA In-Motion." Guides for organizing peer support groups and peer visitation programs also available.


Canadian Diabetes Association
15 Toronto Street, Suite 1001
Toronto, Ontario M5C 2E3 Canada
(416) 363-3373                    In Canada, (800) 226-8464          FAX (416) 214-1899
http://www.diabetes.ca

Provides service and education to individuals with diabetes; serves as an advocate; and provides support for research. Produces a variety of inexpensive educational brochures in English and French. Will mail out reprints of current articles on diabetes and pregnancy.


Centers for Disease Control (CDC)
1600 Clifton Road
Atlanta, GA 30333
(404) 639-3311                    http://www.cdc.gov/nccdphp/ddt/ddthome.htm

The Division of Diabetes Translation conducts research related to the prevalence of diabetes; assesses clinical practices in order to develop optimal treatment; and works with state health departments to develop diabetes control programs.


Diabetes Action Network of the National Federation of the Blind
811 Cherry Street, Suite 309
Columbia, MD 65201
(573) 875-8911

A national support and information network. Publishes a quarterly magazine, "Voice of the Diabetic," which includes personal experiences, medical information, recipes, and resources. Available in standard print and four-track audiocassette. Free. Nonmembers may also obtain free subscriptions but are encouraged to pay $20.00. Also available, "Resource Guide to Aids and Appliances," a list of adaptive equipment; large print, audiocassette, and braille, $2.00.

International Diabetic Athletes Association (IDAA)
1647-B West Bethany Home Road
Phoenix, AZ 85025
(800) 898-4322                    (602) 433-2113                    FAX (602) 433-9331
e-mail: idaa@getnet.com          http://www.getnet.com/~idaa/

An organization that provides education for individuals with diabetes who participate in sports and fitness activities, family members, and service providers through conferences, workshops, and publications. Membership, individuals, $15.00; corporate, $100.00; includes quarterly newsletter, "The Challenge."

Juvenile Diabetes Foundation International (JDF)
The Diabetes Research Foundation
120 Wall Street, 19th Floor
New York, NY 10005
(800) 223-1138                    (212) 889-7575                    FAX (212) 785-9595
e-mail: info@jdfcure.com         http://www.jdfcure.com

JDF Canada:
89 Granton Drive
Richmond Hill, Ontario L4B 2N5 Canada
(905) 889-4171                    FAX (905) 889-4209

Supports research and provides information to individuals with diabetes and their families. Chapters in many states and affiliates in other countries. Annual membership, U.S. and Canada, $25.00, includes quarterly magazine, "Countdown." The World Wide Web site includes an online publication, "Pregnancy and Diabetes."

National Amputation Foundation
73 Church Street
Malverne, NY 11565
(516) 887-3600                    FAX (516) 887-3667

Provides vocational and legal guidance to amputees; produces a variety of inexpensive and free pamphlets. Free publications list. Membership, $25.00.

National Center for Nutrition and Dietetics
American Dietetic Association
216 West Jackson Boulevard
Chicago, IL 60606
Consumer Nutrition Hot-line (800) 366-1655                    (312) 899-0040
FAX (312) 899-1758               http://www.eatright.org

Callers may receive a referral to a registered dietitian or listen to recorded nutrition messages in English and Spanish. Customized food and nutrition information from a registered dietitian is available by calling (900) 225-5267; the cost of a call is $1.95 for the first minute, $.95 for each minute thereafter. Free publications.

National Diabetes Information Clearinghouse (NDIC)
1 Information Way
Bethesda, MD 20892-3560
(301) 654-3327                    FAX (301) 907-8906                    e-mail: ndic@aerie.com

Responds to information requests from the public and professionals. Maintains a database of publications and brochures. Publishes newsletter, "Diabetes Dateline," free. Free list of publications (see "PUBLICATIONS AND TAPES" section below).

National Institute of Diabetes and Digestive and Kidney Diseases (NIDDK)
National Institutes of Health
31 Center Drive, MSC 2560
Building 31, Room 9A-04
Bethesda, MD 20892-2560
(301) 496-3583                    http://www.niddk.nih.gov/

Funds basic and clinical research in the causes, prevention, and treatment of diabetes. Free list of publications. The World Wide Web site contains fact sheets and patient education materials.

National Kidney and Urologic Diseases Information Clearinghouse (NKUDIC)
3 Information Way
Bethesda, MD 20892-3580
(301) 654-4415                    e-mail: nkudic@aerie.com

Responds to individual requests from the public and professionals. Maintains a publications database. Free list of publications.

National Kidney Foundation (NKF)
30 East 33rd Street
New York, NY 10016
(800) 622-9010                    (212) 889-2210

A professional membership organization that provides professional and public education; produces literature on kidney disease; and promotes kidney transplantation and organ donation.

Aerobics for Amputees
Disabled Sports USA (DS/USA)
451 Hungerford Drive, Suite 100
Rockville, Md 20850
(301) 217-0960                    (301) 217-0963 (TT)              FAX (301) 217-0968
e-mail: dsusa@dsusa.org           http://www.dsusa.org/~dsusa/dsusa.html

In this videotape, a person with an amputation demonstrates a specially created exercise routine. 30 minutes. $17.00 plus $4.50 shipping and handling.


Buyer's Guide to Diabetes Products
American Diabetes Association (ADA)
Order Fulfillment
PO Box 930850
Atlanta, GA 31193-0850
(800) 232-6733                    FAX (404) 442-9742

This annual guide compares prices and features for a wide variety of products for people with diabetes. $4.95 plus $3.00 shipping and handling.


Carbohydrate Gram Counter
by Corinne T. Netzer
Distribution Service
Bantam, Doubleday Dell Books
2451 South Wolf Road
Des Plaines, IL 60018

A comprehensive listing of the carbohydrates in fresh foods as well as packaged foods. $4.99 plus $2.50 shipping and handling.


Complete Guide to Diabetes
American Diabetes Association (ADA)
Order Fulfillment
PO Box 930850
Atlanta, GA 31193-0850
(800) 232-6733                    FAX (404) 442-9742

This book includes information about Type I and Type II diabetes, including how to maintain good blood glucose levels, selecting health care providers, planning an exercise program, and enjoying sex. $29.95 plus $3.00 shipping and handling.

Coping with Kidney Failure
by Robert H. Phillips
Avery Publishing Group
120 Old Broadway
Garden City Park, NY 11040
(800) 548-5757                    (516) 741-2155                    FAX (516) 742-1892

This book provides information on kidney dialysis and transplants for individuals with end-stage renal failure. $12.95 plus $3.00 shipping and handling.

Coping with Limb Loss
by Ellen Winchell
Avery Publishing Group
120 Old Broadway
Garden City Park, NY 11040
(800) 548-5757                    (516) 741-2155                    FAX (516) 742-1892

This book provides information about surgery, prosthetics, and rehabilitation as well as practical coping strategies. $14.95 plus $3.00 shipping and handling.

Diabetes and Pregnancy: What to Expect
American Diabetes Association (ADA)
Order Fulfillment
PO Box 930850
Atlanta, GA 31193-0850
(800) 232-6733                    FAX (404) 442-9742

A book with information about insulin therapy, blood glucose monitoring, exercise, and nutrition during pregnancy. $9.95 plus $3.00 shipping and handling.

Diabetes and the Kidneys
American Kidney Fund
6110 Executive Boulevard, Suite 1010
Rockville, MD 20852
(800) 638-8299                    (301) 881-3052                    FAX (301) 881-0898

A booklet that describes how diabetes affects the kidneys' function and measures that may be taken to slow down the course of kidney disease. Free

Diabetes and Vision Loss: Special Considerations
by Marla Bernbaum
in "Meeting the Needs of People with Vision Loss: A Multidisciplinary Perspective"
Resources for Rehabilitation
33 Bedford Street, Suite 19A
Lexington, MA 02173
(617) 862-6455                    FAX (617) 861-7517

Provides information on the psychosocial implications and special rehabilitation needs of individuals with vision loss due to diabetes. Also available on audiocassette. $24.95 plus $5.00 shipping and handling. (See order form on last page of this book.)

Diabetes: Caring for Your Emotions As Well as Your Health
by Jerry Edelwich and Archie Brodsky
Addison-Wesley Publishing Company
1 Jacob Way
Reading, MA 01867
(800) 447-2226                          (617) 944-3700

In addition to describing diabetes and its treatment, this book discusses the many effects diabetes has on social and psychological aspects of life. Practical suggestions for adaptation and relationships with medical personnel and family are provided. Information about sexual function, employment, technology, and support groups is also included. $12.45

Diabetes Self-Management
PO Box 52890
Boulder, CO 80322

A bimonthly magazine that helps people with diabetes manage their disease. Tips on diet, foot care, medical news, etc. U.S., $18.00; Canada, $30.00 (Canadian funds); foreign, $36.00.

The Diabetes Sourcebook
by Diana W. Guthrie and Richard A. Guthrie
Lowell House
Distributed by Contemporary Books Inc.
2 Prudential Plaza, Suite 1200
Chicago, IL 60601
(800) 621-1918                    (312) 540-4500                    FAX (312) 540-4687
Order FAX (800) 998-3103

This book describes diabetes, its complications, psychological issues, and suggestions for management of the disease. Includes information about pregnancy for women with diabetes. $12.95

Diabetes Teaching Guide for People Who Use Insulin
Joslin Diabetes Center
One Joslin Place
Boston, MA 02215
(617) 732-2695                    FAX (617) 732-2562

This book discusses the causes of diabetes, the role of diet and exercise, meal planning, and complications. Also provides information on drawing, mixing, and injecting insulin. $20.00

Diabetes: The Role of Insulin
AIMS Media
9710 DeSoto Avenue
Chatsworth, CA 91311
(800) 367-2467                    (818) 773-4300                    FAX (818) 341-6700

This videotape describes how body cells use insulin and the causes and treatments for hypoglycemia and hyperglycemia.  18 minutes.  $49.95 plus $8.95 shipping and handling.

Diabetes Type II and You and What to Do
by Virginia Valentine, June Biermann, and Barbara Toohey
Lowell House
Distributed by Contemporary Books Inc.
2 Prudential Plaza, Suite 1200
Chicago, IL 60601
(800) 621-1918                    (312) 540-4500                    FAX (312) 540-4687
Order FAX (800) 998-3103

This book describes type II diabetes, diet change, exercise, and emotional aspects.  $11.95

Diabetes, Visual Impairment, and Group Support: A Guidebook
by Judith Caditz
The Center for the Partially Sighted
720 Wilshire Boulevard, Suite 200
Santa Monica, CA 90401-1713
(213) 458-3501                    FAX (310) 458-8179

This guidebook is designed for individuals with diabetes and vision loss, their families, and professionals.  Discusses diabetes mellitus, how it affects vision, psychosocial aspects, diet, assistive devices, and organizing education/support groups.  Standard print and large print.  $12.95 plus $2.50 shipping and handling.

Diabetic Retinopathy: Information for Patients
National Eye Institute (NEI)
Building 31, Room 6A32
Bethesda, MD 20892
(301) 496-5248                    http://www.nei.nih.gov/

This booklet discusses the symptoms of diabetic retinopathy; treatment; vitrectomy; and research. Available free in large print from NEI and on audiocassette ($2.00) from VISION Foundation, Inc., 818 Mt. Auburn Street, Watertown, MA 02172.

The Diabetic Traveler
PO Box 8223 RW
Stamford, CT 06905
(203) 327-5832

A quarterly newsletter that focuses on safe and secure travel; special articles on popular travel destinations. $18.95.

The Diabetic Woman
by Lois Jovanovic-Peterson, June Biermann, and Barbara Toohey
Jeremy Tarcher
Distributed by Putnam Publishing
PO Box 12289
Newark, NJ 07101-5289
(800) 788-6262                    FAX (201) 933-2316

This book focuses on the special issues facing women with diabetes. In addition to generic information about the disease, the book answers questions about menstruation, pregnancy, and sexual relations. Lois Jovanovic-Peterson is a physician who has Type I diabetes; June Biermann has had Type II diabetes since 1965. $13.95 plus $3.50 shipping and handling.

Don't Lose Sight of Diabetic Eye Disease: Information for People at Risk
National Eye Institute (NEI)
Building 31, Room 6A32
Bethesda, MD 20892
(301) 496-5248                    http://www.nei.nih.gov/

This booklet describes how diabetes affects the eyes and problems such as cataract, glaucoma, and diabetic retinopathy. Discusses symptoms, diagnosis, and treatment of diabetic retinopathy. Free in large print from NEI; on audiocassette ($2.00) from VISION Foundation, Inc., 818 Mt. Auburn Street, Watertown, MA 02172.

Exchange Lists for Meal Planning
American Diabetes Association (ADA)
Order Fulfillment
PO Box 930850
Atlanta, GA 31193-0850
(800) 232-6733                    FAX (404) 442-9742

This guide lists foods based on carbohydrate, protein, and fat content. Members, $1.20; nonmembers, $1.50; plus $3.00 shipping and handling. Also available on audiocassette from the National Federation of the Blind, Materials Center, 1800 Johnson Street, Baltimore, MD 21230; $2.00; braille, $10.00.

The Fitness Book: For People with Diabetes
American Diabetes Association (ADA)
Order Fulfillment
PO Box 930850
Atlanta, GA 31193-0850
(800) 232-6733                    FAX (404) 442-9742

This book discusses the benefits of exercise as well as specific exercise programs to control diabetes. $18.95 plus $3.00 shipping and handling.

Gestational Diabetes: What to Expect
American Diabetes Association (ADA)
Order Fulfillment
PO Box 930850
Atlanta, GA 31193-0850
(800) 232-6733                          FAX (404) 442-9742


A book with information about blood glucose monitoring, exercise, and nutrition during pregnancy.
$9.95 plus $3.00 shipping and handling.


A Guide for Women with Diabetes Who Are Pregnant...Or Plan to Be
Joslin Diabetes Center
One Joslin Place
Boston, MA 02215
(617) 732-2695                          FAX (617) 732-2562


This book provides information to help future mothers with optimal nutrition and insulin adjustment
as well as delivery and postpartum care.  $23.50 plus $3.50 shipping and handling.


Know Your Diabetes, Know Yourself
Joslin Diabetes Center
One Joslin Place
Boston, MA  02215
(617) 732-2695                          FAX (617) 732-2562


In this videotape, Joslin patients (not actors) talk about the daily issues of diabetes management: using
a meal plan; the important roles exercise, monitoring, injections, and foot and eye care play in their
lives; and how they manage their disease when sick or traveling.  Joslin health professionals discuss
the essentials of good diabetes care.  60 minutes.  $39.50 plus $3.50 shipping and handling.


Learning to Live Well with Diabetes
by Marion Franz et al.
Chronimed Publishing
13911 Ridgedale Drive, Suite 250
Minnetonka, MN 55343
(800) 848-2793                          In Minneapolis/St. Paul area (612) 546-1146
FAX (800) 395-3003                      FAX in Minneapolis/St. Paul area (612) 541-0739


This collection of articles written by experts addresses current medical treatments and research and
how to live an active life with diabetes.  $24.95 plus $3.00 shipping and handling.


Living with Diabetes  $1.50 per copy
Living with Diabetic Retinopathy  $1.75 per copy
Resources for Rehabilitation
33 Bedford Street, Suite 19A
Lexington, MA 02173
(617) 862-6455                          FAX (617) 861-7517

Designed for distribution by professionals to people with diabetes, these large print (18 point bold type) publications describe the condition, service providers, organizations, devices, and publications. Minimum purchase 25 copies. (See order form on last page of this book.)

Living with Diabetes: A Winning Formula
Info Vision
13425 A Street
Omaha, NE 68144
(800) 237-1808                    FAX (402) 330-9544

This videotape provides information about diet, weight loss, insulin, and self-monitoring of blood glucose and gives recipes. 35 minutes. $25.00 plus $5.00 shipping and handling.

Living with Low Vision: A Resource Guide for People with Sight Loss
Resources for Rehabilitation
33 Bedford Street, Suite 19A
Lexington, MA 02173
(617) 862-6455                    FAX (617) 861-7517

A large print (18 point bold type) comprehensive directory that helps people with sight loss locate the services that they need to remain independent. Chapters describe products that enable people to keep reading, working, and carrying out their daily activities. $43.95 plus $5.00 shipping and handling. (See order form on last page of this book.)

Managing Diabetes on a Budget
American Diabetes Association (ADA)
Order Fulfillment
PO Box 930850
Atlanta, GA 31193-0850
(800) 232-6733                    FAX (770) 442-9742

This book provides advice on finding the best buys on supplies and medications, cooking tips, and general diabetes management. $7.95 plus $3.00 shipping and handling.

Managing Your Gestational Diabetes
by Lois Jovanovic-Peterson with Morton B. Stone
Chronimed Publishing
13911 Ridgedale Drive, Suite 250
Minnetonka, MN 55343
(800) 848-2793                    In Minneapolis/St. Paul area (612) 546-1146
FAX (800) 395-3003               FAX in Minneapolis/St. Paul area (612) 541-0739

This book provides information about controlling diabetes associated with pregnancy and reducing health risks to both the mother and the child. Lois Jovanovic-Peterson is a physician who has diabetes and is a mother herself. $9.95 plus $3.00 shipping and handling.

Monitoring Your Blood Sugar
Juvenile Diabetes Foundation International
The Diabetes Research Foundation
120 Wall Street, 19th Floor
New York, NY 10005
(800) 223-1138                    (212) 889-7575              FAX (212) 785-9595
e-mail: info@jdfcure.com          http://www.jdfcure.com

A brochure that describes the process and benefits of self blood glucose monitoring.  Free

National Diabetes Information Clearinghouse (NDIC)
1 Information Way
Bethesda, MD 20892-3560
(301) 654-3327                    FAX (301) 907-8906                e-mail: ndic@aerie.com

Sponsored by the federal government, this clearinghouse publishes a variety of booklets related to diabetes.  Titles include "The Diabetic Dictionary," a glossary of terms individuals with diabetes are likely to encounter (free); "Noninsulin-Dependent Diabetes" and "Insulin-Dependent Diabetes," two booklets that describes the prevalence, causes, and treatments for each type of diabetes (free); and "The Prevention and Treatment of Five Complications of Diabetes," an overview of the major complications and management of diabetes ($2.00).

National Library Service for the Blind and Physically Handicapped (NLS)
1291 Taylor Street, NW
Washington, DC 20542
(800) 424-8567 or 8572 (Reference Section)
(800) 424-9100 (to receive application)
(202) 707-5100                    FAX (202) 707-0712
telnet marvel.loc.gov  (log in as marvel, select Library of Congress Online Systems, select connect to LOCIS, then select "Braille and Audio" for a catalogue of braille and tape publications)

Serves individuals in the U.S. and U.S. residents living abroad through a network of regional libraries.  Individuals must be unable to read standard print due to visual impairment or physical disability.  "Facts: Books for Blind and Physically Handicapped Individuals" describes NLS programs and eligibility requirements.  Order form lists general information brochures, magazines and newsletters, directories, reference circulars, and subject and reference bibliographies.  "Talking Book Topics," published bimonthly in large print, audiocassette, and disc, lists titles recently added to the national collection which are available through the network of regional libraries.  All services and publications from NLS are free.

Rehabilitation Resource Manual: VISION
Resources for Rehabilitation
33 Bedford Street, Suite 19A
Lexington, MA 02173
(617) 862-6455                    FAX (617) 861-7517

A desk reference that enables professionals to make effective referrals.  Includes chapters on breaking the news of irreversible vision loss; guidelines on starting self-help groups; information on research and professional organizations; plus chapters on services and products for special population groups and by eye conditions and diseases. $39.95 plus $5.00 shipping and handling. (See order form on last page of this book.)

The Sun, the Rain and the Insulin
by Joan MacCracken
Tiffin Press of Maine
PO Box 549
Orono, ME 04473-0549

This book portrays the lives of six families who have a member with diabetes. Set in a family camp for people with diabetes, the families discuss their concerns, their frustrations, and their solutions to problems that arise in the management of diabetes. $12.95 plus $2.00 shipping and handling.

Take Charge of Your Diabetes
Centers for Disease Control (CDC)
1600 Clifton Road
Atlanta, GA 30333
(404) 488-5020                     http://www.cdc.gov/nccdphp/ddt/ddthome.htm

A book written in simple language to help people with diabetes manage their disease. Information on blood sugar, dental, foot, vision, and kidney problems, and nerve damage. Includes forms for keeping records of visits with health care providers and sick days. Free

Taking Charge of Your Diabetes
Unitech Communications
9500 Euclid Avenue, KK 11
Cleveland, OH 44195-5020
FAX (216) 721-7678

In this videotape, specialists describe diabetes management techniques, suggest questions to ask physicians, and discuss doctor-patient relationships. 60 minutes. $19.95. Also available, "Your Diabetes Guide," a manual that reviews nutrition, blood sugar and urine testing, and exercise as diabetes management techniques. Lists resources such as newsletters, organizations, journals, and cookbooks. $24.95

A Touch of Diabetes
by Lois Jovanovic-Peterson, Charles M. Peterson, and Morton Stone
Chronimed Publishing
13911 Ridgedale Drive, Suite 250
Minnetonka, MN 55343
(800) 848-2793                     In Minneapolis/St. Paul area (612) 546-1146
FAX (800) 395-3003                 FAX in Minneapolis/St. Paul area (612) 541-0739

This guide to help people with Type II diabetes manage their condition includes information about preventing complications and dietary advice. $10.95 plus $3.00 shipping and handling.

Type II Diabetes: Your Healthy Living Guide
American Diabetes Association (ADA)
Order Fulfillment
PO Box 930850
Atlanta, GA 31193-0850
(800) 232-6733                    FAX (404) 442-9742

A guidebook that helps people with Type II diabetes manage their disease through proper diet, exercise, and the safe use of medications. $24.95 plus $3.00 shipping and handling.

# Chapter 6

# *EPILEPSY*

Epilepsy is a condition in which the brain's cells undergo abnormal electrical activity, causing disturbances in the nervous system. An epileptic seizure occurs when there is an excessive discharge of electrical impulses from these nerve cells. To be classified as epilepsy, these seizures must be recurring events. Individuals who have isolated incidents of seizures do not have epilepsy. Epilepsy is not a single disease or condition, nor is it contagious. It often develops in people whose families have no history of epilepsy, although children of individuals with epilepsy are thought to have a greater chance of developing this condition (Epilepsy Foundation of America: 1993).

Although most studies indicate that epilepsy is somewhat more prevalent in men than women (Kurtz: 1991), the condition can be very serious for women of childbearing age and for their fetuses. Yerby (1991) states that 40% of all Americans with epilepsy, or 800,000 women, are potential mothers. The onset of epilepsy often coincides with puberty and the beginning of menstruation in girls and is related to the hormones produced by the reproductive system (Kurtz: 1991). Epilepsy is the most common neurological disorder of pregnancy, occurring in one out of 200 pregnancies (Morrison and Rieder: 1993).

In order to diagnose their specific type of epileptic seizures and syndromes, women are often asked to come to the physician's office with a family member or other individual who has witnessed their seizures. Patients, family members, or friends should provide the physician with a detailed description of the seizure activity, including onset, frequency, any changes in the seizures, duration, and medication usage. Severe head trauma, stroke, and infections in the central nervous system are the greatest risks for epilepsy. When an individual over age 20 has a seizure for the first time, a brain tumor should be suspected (Epilepsy Foundation of America: 1992).

The electroencephalograph (EEG) is used to determine where in the brain the seizure activity is taking place. Sometimes the EEG does not pick up the brain's electrical changes, or the woman may not experience any seizure activity while being monitored. In some instances, a woman may be hospitalized so that a 24 hour EEG recording may be made. Blood tests and tests of spinal fluid are conducted to determine if an infection has caused the seizure. Computerized tomography scans (CTs) or magnetic resonance imaging (MRIs) may be performed to detect the presence of tumors, scar tissue, or blood clots that could be the cause of seizures.

Some individuals with epilepsy who are candidates for surgery are participating in research to locate areas of abnormal brain metabolism. Positron emission tomography (PET) allows researchers to observe the brain's metabolic activity by measuring the brain's use of glucose, oxygen, and carbon dioxide. Positron emission tomography may also reveal the effects of antiepileptic drugs (National Institute of Neurological Disorders and Stroke: 1984).

## *TYPES OF SEIZURES*

*Generalized seizures* affect both hemispheres of the brain and may lead to loss of consciousness, convulsions, and loss of memory. Two types of generalized seizures are the tonic-clonic and absence seizures.

A *tonic-clonic seizure* (previously called a grand mal seizure) is a generalized seizure with loss of consciousness. The individual may cry out, fall, and lie rigid. The woman's body may jerk, and she may lose bladder and bowel control. She may bite her tongue, and saliva may appear around the mouth. When the woman regains consciousness, she may feel sore or stiff. She may or may not have any warning of the impending episode. She will not remember the seizure, and she may experience a headache and drowsiness, sometimes taking several days to return to her normal functioning (Dichter: 1994).

An *absence seizure* (previously called a petit mal seizure) is characterized by sudden onset and a blank stare. These seizures last a short time but may occur many times a day, beginning and ending abruptly. The individual is unaware of her surroundings and may not respond when spoken to, although sometimes speaking to her will stop the absence seizure.

If only one hemisphere of the brain is affected, the seizure is called a *partial* (or *focal*) *seizure*. Symptoms of a partial seizure include an involuntary turning of the head, loss of speech, sweating, pallor, dilation of the pupils, and light flashes. Tingling or numbness in the face or fingers or hearing buzzing noises may also occur. Individuals do not lose consciousness during a partial seizure.

*Complex partial seizures*, which sometimes affect the temporal lobes (at the side of the brain near the ears), can also occur in several other areas of the brain. Women having a complex partial seizure appear to be in a trance accompanied by involuntary motor activities, called automatisms. They lose consciousness and have no control over these movements, which may include lip and tongue smacking, mimicry, hand movements, or repetitive utterances.

The individual is conscious during a *simple partial seizure,* but she cannot control body movements. An arm or leg may jerk or tremble. Seizure activity occurs in the part of the brain which controls vision, hearing, sensation, or memory. She may feel disoriented or fearful, or she may experience odd sensations on one side of the body.

An *aura* is an unusual feeling experienced by many people with epilepsy prior to a seizure. The individual may feel sick or apprehensive, have aural or visual hallucinations, or notice a peculiar odor or taste. The individual retains memory of the sensation even if she loses consciousness. The aura often serves as a warning that a seizure is about to take place, allowing her to move away from potential hazards before the onset of a major seizure.

## *TREATMENT OF EPILEPSY*

Most individuals with epilepsy use antiepileptic drugs to control seizures. The choice of antiepileptic drug is determined by the type of seizure, other clinical aspects of the seizure, the drug's side effects, cost, and method of administration. Smith (1990) recommends that drug therapy begin with a single antiepileptic drug, although the individual experiencing more than one type of seizure may need more than one drug to gain control of the seizures. Drugs such as carbamazepine (Tegretol), phenobarbital (Luminal and others) and phenytoin (Dilantin) are used to treat tonic-clonic seizures; valproic acid (Depakene, Depakote) is effective in treating a variety of seizures (Brodie and Dichter: 1996). Blood tests are used to monitor the efficacy of the chosen drug.

It is important for women with epilepsy to maintain a fixed schedule for taking medication. Missing a dose, ceasing to take medication, or taking the wrong dosage may lead to seizure activity. Women taking antiepileptic medication should tell physicians treating them for other conditions about their epilepsy medicine and inquire about interactions with both over-the-counter products and prescription drugs. Two-thirds of the individuals who are treated successfully with antiepileptic drugs may be weaned off these medications (Brodie and Dichter: 1996).

Side effects of antiepileptic drugs may include nausea, fatigue, slurring of words, staggering, or allergic reactions (a rash or hives). Some women experience emotional changes, while others may note memory, learning, or behavior problems. Effects on appearance are not uncommon, including alopecia (hair loss) and weight gain (McGuire: 1991). Women should ask the physician about each drug's side effects and what to do if a reaction occurs.

Experimental drugs are available through special testing programs at medical epilepsy centers. The Epilepsy Foundation of America will direct individuals to a local center (see "ORGANIZATIONS" section below).

Surgery may be considered when the seizures always originate in one part of the brain; if medication has been unsuccessful; or when surgery will not affect vision, speech, movement, or memory. In resective surgery, the portion of the brain that causes the seizures is removed. In an anterior temporal lobectomy, the front or anterior part of one of the temporal lobes is removed in order to reduce partial seizures. Individuals with partial and generalized seizures may undergo surgery to interrupt the nerve pathways by cutting into the hemispheres of the brain in a procedure called a corpus callostomy (Devinsky: 1994). Individuals considering surgery must understand that although surgical procedures may reduce the number and frequency of seizures, most individuals will still require medication to bring remaining seizure activity under control (Gumnit: 1995).

Tyler (1990) believes that surgery is not considered as often as it should be because the danger of such surgery is overestimated and the benefits underestimated. In addition, family physicians sometimes lack knowledge of specialized epilepsy surgery centers. The National Institute of Neurological Disorders and Stroke (1988) reports that more than 100,000 individuals with partial seizures who do not respond to medical therapy are candidates for surgery. Women should ask physicians about the risks and benefits of surgery in their own situation. If a physician cannot supply the information, women should ask for a referral to another specialist or contact the National Institute of Neurological Disorders and Stroke for information on surgical procedures. Brain surgery should never be undertaken without serious investigation into the pro's and con's. Talking with other women who have chosen surgery and those who have not may help the woman make the best possible decision for her health.

## EPILEPSY IN OLDER WOMEN

Seizures in older women may be the result of systemic illness; the use of medications such as analgesics and antihistamines; or the withdrawal of sedative drugs. The incidence of epilepsy increases in later life, with nearly 20% of newly diagnosed cases of epilepsy occurring in postmenopausal women (Usiskin: 1991). It is crucial to identify any primary medical conditions that may precipitate seizures. Examples of systemic illnesses which may cause seizure activity include strokes (which may cause acute seizures followed by recurring seizure activity) and either primary or metastatic brain tumors. Once seizures symptomatic of systemic illness have been distinguished from epilepsy, they should be treated by managing the precipitating event without the use of antiepileptic drugs (Troupin and Johannessen: 1990).

Antiepileptic drugs affect the supply of calcium to an older woman's bones, contributing to the development of osteoporosis. Consequently they are more vulnerable to fractures if a seizure results in a fall. Tonic-clonic seizures pose additional problems for elders who also have heart or pulmonary disease. Stress on the heart, pain, or breathing problems are potential aftereffects of such seizures (Devinsky: 1994).

Older women with chronic epilepsy may be affected by pharmacologic changes, such as changes in metabolism related to the aging process, and may require adjustment in their usual seizure therapy. Side effects of medication, such as balance problems, confusion, and drowsiness, may put them at risk for falls. Because older women often take drugs for a variety of conditions, those with epilepsy must be concerned about the interaction of these drugs and antiepileptic drugs. Women should be certain to ask their physicians about the possible interaction among the various drugs they are taking.

# SEXUAL FUNCTIONING

In the past, individuals with epilepsy were forbidden by law to marry, due to false beliefs about the role of heredity and mental function. Now that there is a better understanding of epilepsy, these laws no longer exist. Marriage and childbearing rates in women with epilepsy do not differ from those for women without epilepsy (Epilepsy Foundation of America: 1987).

In some individuals, epilepsy reduces libido and therefore sexual activity. Women with epilepsy may fear close relationships, because they do not feel comfortable disclosing their condition. Some women may fear that sexual activity will cause seizures and that the seizures will be detrimental to their sexual relations. Usiskin (1991) reports that some women confuse the physical characteristics of a seizure with orgasm. Although talking about epilepsy may be difficult at first, it is important to inform anyone who spends time with the woman, including sexual partners, about the condition and what to do if a seizure occurs.

## FAMILY PLANNING, PREGNANCY, AND CHILDREARING

Women who choose oral contraceptives for birth control should tell their physicians if they take antiepileptic drugs. Certain antiepileptic drugs, such as phenobarbital, impair the effectiveness of birth control pills. The physician should recommend an oral contraceptive that will be most effective for birth control while still taking measures to prevent seizure activity. Since 1991 another method of contraception available in this country is Norplant, the implantation of a synthetic progesterone that prevents ovulation for as long as five years. Although side effects are minimal, women who take certain antiepileptic drugs such as Dilantin or Tegretol are advised against using Norplant (Murphy: 1993). Recently, women have filed suit against the manufacturer of Norplant for pain and scarring associated with its removal. Fertility rates are reduced in women with epilepsy, especially in those who have complex partial seizures (Kurtz: 1991).

At least 90% of women with epilepsy who are treated with antiepileptic drugs deliver infants with no birth defects (Epilepsy Foundation of America: 1990). However, pregnancy in women with epilepsy is considered high risk and requires special management by neurologists and obstetricians. Women with epilepsy who plan to become pregnant should discuss their medications with their physician prior to conception. If they wait until after conception, the fetus may already have fully formed organs and the opportunity to alter drug therapy may have passed (Crawford: 1993). Since all antiepileptic drugs have been implicated in an increase in birth defects, and some cause developmental delays of the central nervous system (Morrison and Rieder: 1993), prepregnancy counseling should include a discussion of the risk factors for both mother and child.

The probability of prematurity, neonatal and perinatal* death, stillbirth, and hemorrhage in the fetus is higher for women with epilepsy than for women who do not have epilepsy (Crawford: 1993). The risk of birth defects is two to three times higher for the children of women with epilepsy who are taking medication to control seizures than for women who do not have epilepsy. Birth defects are one to two times more frequent in the children of women with epilepsy who are not taking seizure medication than in the children of women who do not have epilepsy (Epilepsy Foundation of America: 1991). The most common birth defects are cleft lip, cleft palate, and congenital heart conditions. Women who take antiepileptic drugs such as valproate and carbamazepine, a commonly prescribed drug for epilepsy management despite recent controversy over its safety during pregnancy (Morrison

*shortly before and after birth, usually defined as the 29th week of gestation until 4 weeks after birth

and Rieder: 1993), have a higher risk of delivering a child with spina bifida (Treiman: 1993). Ultrasound tests may detect the presence of this congenital malformation.

Seizures are likely to increase in frequency during pregnancy in a large proportion of mothers. There is some debate over the ability to predict increased frequency of seizures. While Montouris and colleagues (1979) indicate that frequency of seizures during the two years prior to pregnancy is a good predictor of seizures during pregnancy, Yerby (1991) states that it is difficult to predict which women will be likely to have increased seizures, as they are not related to type of epilepsy, its duration, or seizures during previous pregnancies. However, it is known that there is greater risk to the fetus for mothers who have seizures during pregnancy than those who do not. Some mothers deliberately reduce the dosage of their antiepileptic drugs during pregnancy because of their fears of the drugs' effect on the fetus, and therefore may be subject to having seizures. It is known that the metabolic changes that occur during pregnancy cause the antiepileptic drugs to be less effective, even when their dosage remains constant. If the mother has a seizure while pregnant and her breathing is affected, a lack of oxygen to the fetus may be a concern; if she falls, she may also cause harm to herself and to the fetus. Mothers who experience tonic-clonic seizures are especially at risk for falling. These generalized seizures may result in the suppression of fetal heart beat, and, less commonly, miscarriage. Partial seizures do not present the same risk unless they become generalized to the whole brain (Yerby: 1991).

If a woman has been seizure free for years, she and her physician may decide to decrease antiepileptic drugs gradually over a period of time before she conceives. If this strategy is not possible due to seizure activity, the use of a single antiepileptic drug in the lowest effective dose to maintain seizure control is recommended (International League Against Epilepsy: 1993).

Some women develop their first seizures during pregnancy, a condition called gestational epilepsy. Three-quarters of these women will have seizures after pregnancy; many of these women have vascular abnormalities or tumors which are activated by the changes that occur during pregnancy (Montouris et al.: 1979).

Women should be carefully monitored during pregnancy and may expect to require some adjustment in antiepileptic medication. Infants born to mothers with epilepsy who take certain antiepileptic drugs may develop hemorrhagic disease due to an insufficient levels of vitamin K. This disorder may be prevented by the administration of vitamin K to the mother prior to delivery and to the newborn after delivery. Blood clotting studies should be performed to ensure that clotting times have become normal. Babies born to mothers who have taken barbiturates such as phenobarbital to control seizure activity during pregnancy may exhibit excessive sleepiness or drug withdrawal after delivery.

Crawford (1993) reports that children whose mothers have epilepsy are more likely to develop the condition than those whose fathers have epilepsy. The risks are greater if both parents or other family members have epilepsy. A genetics specialist can offer information on risks, based on the family's epilepsy history. The fact remains, however, that most women with epilepsy give birth to children who do not develop the condition.

If the mother is not free of seizures, it is important that she have sufficient assistance with child care to avoid seizure related accidents to both herself and the child. A mother may choose bottle feeding over breastfeeding so that this duty can be shared with a partner or child care assistant. The lack of sleep encountered by new mothers may trigger a seizure. Women who experience an aura or another warning sign prior to a seizure should consider using a personal emergency response system to summon help before they lose consciousness. A woman who adapted her child care patterns describes them as follows:

> As a mother with frequent seizures, I was very concerned for the baby,
> but I managed to keep things simple. When he cried, I'd hold him while
> sitting on the floor. That's how I fed and changed him, too. I'd wait to
> bathe him until my husband was home. Then we'd both give him a bath,
> which was fun. (Epilepsy Foundation of America: 1996)

In addition to these suggestions, women should also consider wearing a medical identification bracelet indicating that they have epilepsy so that emergency assistance may be provided appropriately.

Seeing their mother experience a seizure can be very frightening to children. As soon as they are old enough to understand, parents should explain the mother's condition to their children. Children should learn how to summon help if their mother has a seizure and what they can do to help her. Most telephones may be pre-programmed for emergency calls to fire, police, and rescue squads. Usiskin (1991) describes how she taught her own children to cope with her seizures by assigning them each a role, such as placing a cloth under her face to prevent abrasion. Learning that their mother is not in pain during the seizures can be very comforting information for the children.

## PSYCHOLOGICAL ASPECTS OF EPILEPSY

Various studies have concluded that depression is more common among people with epilepsy than among the general population. Although these studies have been conducted by psychiatrists, neurologists, and general practitioners, they are all remarkably consistent in reaching this conclusion (Robertson: 1991).

The diagnosis of epilepsy is difficult to accept:

> Some individuals are more disabled by the fact that they have epilepsy
> than by the seizures themselves and unduly restrict their activities or
> withdraw from social interactions (Dichter: 1994, 2233).

Depression in women with epilepsy may be due to the stresses of living with epilepsy; employment problems; or the inability to drive. They may complain of fatigue or feeling sad; may sleep poorly; or may be unable to concentrate. These symptoms may be related to having epilepsy, or they may signal a problem with medication. Masland (1985) found that disability in individuals with epilepsy was related to the disruption caused by the seizures; the effects of associated neurological impairments, including those caused by drugs; reactions of society; and the individual's self-concept.

Snyder's study (1990) of individuals age 18 or over who had had epilepsy for at least one year found that the need to take medications regularly and not knowing when a seizure would occur caused the greatest amount of stress. Ostracism, which has often been cited as a cause of stress, was not a high stressor for these subjects. Individuals who ranked their health as good were more likely to take measures to control their health than were subjects who ranked their health as poor; such measures included relaxation techniques and biofeedback, although the efficacy of these measures is not known.

Upton (1993) reports that perceived support from both family and friends was a factor in the emotional adjustment of individuals with epilepsy. He also found that gender was unrelated to social support or emotional adjustment. Upton and Thompson (1992) found that those subjects who used "wish fulfilling fantasies" as a coping mechanism, that is they wished for a miracle that would cure them, had low levels of self-esteem and acceptance of the condition and high levels of anxiety and depression. Those who coped through "cognitive restructuring," finding positive aspects to the condition such as developing inner strength, were most likely to accept the condition and have lower

156

levels of anxiety, depression, and social avoidance. Participating in a self-help group or discussing negative feelings with a physician, psychologist, or social worker may be helpful. Some people also use stress reduction and relaxation techniques.

Unemployment and underemployment are among the most serious social problems of individuals with epilepsy. It is important that employers understand the effects of epilepsy and antiepileptic drugs. Although unpredictable seizures are hazardous in certain environments, they are less significant than the ignorance and fear of employers and employees. It is equally important that unfounded myths and stereotypes be confronted so that women with epilepsy have the opportunity they deserve in the workplace. However, it is often difficult for them to choose when to disclose their condition. Poor self-image may have a negative effect on the skills necessary to seek employment and interpersonal relationships. The combination of self-stigma, perceived and actual societal stigma, and the lack of social skills and confidence leads to a tendency to blame epilepsy for every failure in life.

The lack of a driver's license can be a significant barrier to employment, activities of everyday living, and social life for women with epilepsy. In most states, individuals must be free of seizures for six months to one year in order to be eligible for a driver's license. A letter from a physician which states that seizures are under control may be required.

It is often difficult for women with epilepsy to purchase health, life, or automobile insurance. Even when insurance is available, the premiums may be very high or exclusions may be made for claims relating to epilepsy.

## *PROFESSIONAL SERVICE PROVIDERS*

Women who experience a seizure will first see a ***primary care physician***. Hospitalization may be required to observe the individual for progressive symptoms or additional seizures. An outpatient visit may be sufficient if the seizure occurred more than a week before medical consultation and was an isolated event. The primary care physician may initiate treatment at this time.

If initial treatment does not achieve seizure control in about three months, a woman should be referred to a ***neurologist*** for a thorough evaluation. A neurologist is a physician who diagnoses and treats conditions involving the brain and nervous system, including epilepsy. A ***neurosurgeon*** performs any necessary brain surgery.

If seizures are not under control within nine months of treatment, referral to a comprehensive treatment center is recommended. The National Association of Epilepsy Centers has established guidelines for these specialized epilepsy treatment centers (Gumnit: 1990). Women who wish to become pregnant should be treated jointly by their neurologist and their ***obstetrician***. Together these physicians and the woman can develop a plan to manage seizures and to protect the health of the woman and her fetus.

***Social workers*** provide information about financial and medical benefits, housing, and community resources. They conduct individual, family, or group counseling and may refer individuals to self-help or peer counseling groups.

***Rehabilitation counselors*** coordinate services such as vocational rehabilitation, education, and training for women with epilepsy. The rehabilitation counselor can serve as an advocate with prospective employers who may be uninformed or fearful about hiring an individual with epilepsy. Women with epilepsy who are unemployed or underemployed should apply to their state vocational rehabilitation agency for assistance with career planning, training, and placement.

Physicians who treat people with epilepsy are often located in private practices. Women who live in metropolitan areas will find neurological clinics and comprehensive epilepsy centers available at major hospitals or universities. Comprehensive epilepsy centers and programs around the country provide medical care; conduct multidisciplinary research; train physicians, nurses, and other caregivers; and help to organize community services. They are usually affiliated with university medical centers and serve a designated geographic area. The Epilepsy Foundation of America will refer individuals to local affiliates.

## *ENVIRONMENTAL ADAPTATIONS*

Women whose seizures are under control have no restrictions on their recreational activities. However, it is important to take extra precautions with activities such as swimming, waterskiing, scuba, and sky diving, since the occurrence of a seizure is very dangerous while engaged in these activities. It is a good idea for women to wear an identification bracelet or necklace or carry a wallet card which indicates that they have epilepsy. When traveling, it is wise to carry a letter from a physician describing the seizure disorder and medications currently used. A medication routine may need to be adjusted when travel affects sleep schedules.

Personal safety should be considered in everyday activities. Lowering the temperature of the water and sitting down to shower may prevent injury if a seizure occurs while bathing. Wall-to-wall carpeting and padding on sharp corners reduce the risk of injury in falls. In the kitchen, using appliances such as food processors and blenders lowers the risk of injuries due to sharp knives. Using a microwave oven reduces burns and substituting plastic cups and dishes prevents cuts when a seizure occurs. Safety gates at the top of staircases; automatic shut-off switches on appliances such as irons, power tools, and lawnmowers; and barriers in front of fireplaces, hot radiators, and heaters, will also prevent injuries.

## *HOW TO RECOGNIZE A SEIZURE AND GIVE FIRST AID*

Epileptic seizures have been mistakenly identified as heart attacks, drunkenness, and drug overdoses. It is important for all health professionals, rehabilitation professionals, and the general public to recognize epileptic seizures and to know simple first aid for epilepsy.
- Remove hard or sharp items that are in the vicinity.
- Loosen the collar to make breathing easier.
- Place a flat, soft cushion, folded jacket, or sweater under the individual's head.
- Gently turn her head to the side to help keep the airway clear. Do not try to place any object between the teeth of anyone experiencing a seizure.
- Do not try to stop her jerking movements.
- Check to see if she is wearing an identification bracelet or necklace or carrying an identification card which states that she has epilepsy.
- Remain with her until the seizure ends and offer assistance, if needed.
- If she seems confused, offer to call a family member, friend, or taxi to help her get home.
- If the seizure continues for more than five minutes, if another seizure begins shortly after the first, or if she does not regain consciousness after the jerking movements have ceased, call an ambulance. If she has other medical conditions

such as heart disease or diabetes or she is pregnant, it is also wise to call an ambulance.

• If the individual is having an absence seizure, she may have a dazed appearance, stare into space, or exhibit automatic behavior such as shaking an arm or leg. Speak quietly and calmly and move her away from any dangerous areas, such as a flight of stairs or a stove. Remain with her until she regains consciousness.

## References

Brodie, Martin J. and Marc A. Dichter
1996   "Antiepileptic Drugs" The New England Journal of Medicine 335(January):3:168-175
Crawford, Pamela
1993   "Epilepsy and Pregnancy" Seizure 2:87-90
Devinsky, Orrin
1994   A Guide to Understanding and Living with Epilepsy Philadelphia, PA: F.A. Davis Company
Dichter, Mark A.
1994   "The Epilepsies and Convulsive Disorders" pp. 2223-2244 in Kurt J. Isselbacher et al. (eds.) Harrison's Principles of Internal Medicine New York, NY: McGraw Hill
Epilepsy Foundation of America
1996   Safety and Seizures Landover, MD: Epilepsy Foundation of America
1993   Questions and Answers About Epilepsy Landover, MD: Epilepsy Foundation of America
1992   Seizure Recognition and Observation Landover, MD: Epilepsy Foundation of America
1991   Epilepsy in Pregnancy Landover, MD: Epilepsy Foundation of America
1990   Medicines for Epilepsy Landover, MD: Epilepsy Foundation of America
1987   Epilepsy: Part of Your Life Landover, MD: Epilepsy Foundation of America
Gumnit, Robert J.
1995   Your Child and Epilepsy New York, NY: Demos Vermande
1990   "Interplay of Economics, Politics, and Quality in the Care of Patients with Epilepsy: The Formation of the National Association of Epilepsy Centers" Appendix I in Dennis B. Smith (ed.) Epilepsy: Current Approaches to Diagnosis and Treatment New York, NY: Raven Press
International League Against Epilepsy, Commission on Genetics, Pregnancy and the Child
1993   "Guidelines for the Care of Women of Childbearing Age with Epilepsy" Epilepsia 34(4):588-589
Kurtz, Zarrina
1991   "Sex Differences in Epilepsy: Epidemiological Aspects" in Michael R. Trimble (ed.) Women and Epilepsy Chichester, England: John Wiley & Sons
Masland, R. L.
1985   "Psychosocial Aspects of Epilepsy" pp. 357-377 in Roger J. Porter (ed.) The Epilepsies Stoneham, MA: Butterworth-Heineman
McGuire, A. M.
1991   "Quality of Life in Women with Epilepsy" pp. 13-30 in Michael R. Trimble (ed.) Women and Epilepsy Chichester, England: John Wiley & Sons
Montouris, Georgia D., Gerald M. Fenichel, and L. William McLain
1979   "The Pregnant Epileptic: A Review and Recommendations" Archives of Neurology 36-(October):601-603

Morrison, C. and M. J. Rieder

1993 "Practices of Epilepsy during Pregnancy: A Survey of Canadian Neurologists" <u>Reproductive Toxicology</u> 7:1:55-59

Murphy, Eileen

1993 "Norplant: A New Birth Control Option for Women with Disabilities" <u>Resourceful Woman</u> 2(Fall)3:1,5

National Institute of Neurological Disorders and Stroke

1988 <u>The Surgical Management of Epilepsy</u> Bethesda, MD: National Institute of Neurological Disorders and Stroke

1984 <u>Positron Emission Tomography: Emerging Research Opportunities in the Neurosciences</u> Bethesda, MD: National Institute of Neurological Disorders and Stroke

Robertson, Mary M.

1991 "Depression in Epilepsy" pp. 223-242 in Michael R. Trimble (ed.) <u>Women and Epilepsy</u> Chichester, England: John Wiley & Sons

Smith, Dennis B.

1990 "Antiepileptic Drug Selection in Adults" pp. 111-138 in Dennis B. Smith (ed.) <u>Epilepsy: Current Approaches to Diagnosis and Treatment</u> New York, NY: Raven Press

Snyder, Mariah

1990 "Stressors, Coping Mechanisms, and Perceived Health in Persons with Epilepsy" <u>International Disability Studies</u> 12:3:100-103

Treiman, D.M.

1993 "Current Treatment Strategies in Selected Situations in Epilepsy" <u>Epilepsia</u> 34 Suppl 5:S17-23

Troupin, Alan S. and Svein I. Johannessen

1990 "Epilepsy in the Elderly" pp. 141-153 in Dennis B. Smith (ed.) <u>Epilepsy: Current Approaches to Diagnosis and Treatment</u> New York, NY: Raven Press

Tyler, Allen R.

1990 "The Role of Surgery in Therapy for Epilepsy" pp. 173-182 in Dennis B. Smith (ed.) <u>Epilepsy: Current Approaches to Diagnosis and Treatment</u> New York, NY: Raven Press

Upton, Dominic

1993 "Social Support and Emotional Adjustment in People with Chronic Epilepsy" <u>Journal of Epilepsy</u> 6:2:105-111

Upton, Dominic and Pamela J. Thompson

1992 "Effectiveness of Coping Strategies Employed by People with Chronic Epilepsy" <u>Journal of Epilepsy</u> 5:2:119-127

Usiskin, Susan C.

1991 "The Woman with Epilepsy" pp. 3-12 in Michael R. Trimble (ed.) <u>Women and Epilepsy</u> Chichester, England: John Wiley & Sons

Yerby, Mark S.

1991 "Pregnancy and Teratogenesis" pp. 167-192 in Michael R. Trimble (ed.) <u>Women and Epilepsy</u> Chichester, England: John Wiley & Sons

AED (Antiepileptic Drug) Pregnancy Registry
Massachusetts General Hospital
Fruit Street
Boston, MA 02114
(888) 233-2334                    (617) 726-1742                    FAX (617) 724-1911
e-mail: huntington@helix.mgh.harvard.edu
http://neuro-www2.mgh.harvard.edu/aed/registry.nclk

This project is recruiting women who are taking antiepileptic drugs for an epidemiological study of the effects of the drugs on the health of their children.


Brain Injury Association
1776 Massachusetts Avenue, NW, Suite 100
Washington, DC 20036
Family Helpline (800) 444-6443        (202) 296-6443                    FAX (202) 296-8850

A membership organization that provides information and support for individuals with head injury, their families, and professionals. (Seizures are often precipitated by a head injury.) Local affiliates. Membership, $35.00, includes quarterly newsletter, "TBI Challenge!" and discounts on publications, conferences, and seminars. A reduced rate of $5.00 is available to persons with brain injury or family members who have limited resources. Also publishes the "National Directory of Brain Injury Rehabilitation Services." Members, $40.00; nonmembers, $45.00; plus $5.00 shipping and handling. "Catalogue of Educational Materials," free; plus $2.00 shipping.


Epilepsy Foundation of America (EFA)
4351 Garden City Drive, Suite 406
Landover, MD 20785
(800) 332-1000                    (800) 332-2070 (TT)              (301) 459-3700
FAX (301) 577-2684                (301) 577-0100 (telephone orders only)
e-mail: postmaster@efa.org        http://www.efa.org

Provides information and education, advocacy, research support, and services to individuals with epilepsy, their family members, and professionals. Some publications and audio-visual materials are available in Spanish. Membership, $25.00, includes low-cost medication program, 10% discount on publications and videotapes, and monthly newsletter, "Epilepsy USA." Limited membership, $5.00, provides eligibility for prescription drug program only. Local affiliates.


National Association of Epilepsy Centers (NAEC)
5775 Wayzata Boulevard, Suite 225
Minneapolis, MN 55416
(612) 525-4526                    FAX (612) 525-1560

An organization of epilepsy centers that helps to develop standards for medical and surgical treatment of epilepsy and for the facilities and programs that serve individuals with epilepsy. The NAEC also advises government and industry officials about the needs of people with epilepsy and offers technical assistance to the centers serving these individuals.

National Easter Seal Society
230 West Monroe Street, Suite 1800
Chicago, IL 60606
(800) 221-6827                (312) 726-6200                (312) 726-4258 (TT)
FAX (312) 726-1494           e-mail: nessinfo@seals.com     http://www.seals.com

Provides information and services to individuals with epilepsy, their families, and professionals. Local affiliates.

National Epilepsy Library
Epilepsy Foundation of America (EFA)
4351 Garden City Drive, Suite 406
Landover, MD 20785
(800) 332-4050                (301) 459-3700                FAX (301) 577-2684
e-mail: postmaster@efa.org    http://www.efa.org

A professional library for physicians and other health professionals. Maintains database of articles and publications on medical and psychosocial aspects of epilepsy. Distributes "Quarterly Update," a bibliography of newly acquired resources. Free

National Institute of Neurological Disorders and Stroke (NINDS)
Building 31, Room 8A06
31 Center Drive, MSC 2540
Bethesda, MD 20892-2540
(800) 352-9424               (301) 496-5751                FAX (301) 402-2186
http://www.ninds.nih.gov

Supports clinical and basic research, maintains national specimen banks for the study of brain and other tissue, and publishes professional and public education materials.

National Stroke Association
96 Inverness Drive East, Suite I
Englewood, Colorado 80112-5112
(800) 787-6537               (303) 649-9299                FAX (303) 649-1328
e-mail: info@stroke.org      http://www.stroke.org

Assists individuals with stroke and educates their families, physicians, and the general public about stroke and the risk of seizures. Membership, $20.00, includes quarterly newsletter, "Be Stroke Smart," and discount on publications.

Women and Epilepsy Initiative
Epilepsy Foundation of America (EFA)
4351 Garden City Drive, Suite 406
Landover, MD 20785
(800) 332-1000                    (800) 332-2070 (TT)              (301) 459-3700
FAX (301) 577-2684               (301) 577-0100 (telephone orders only)
e-mail: postmaster@efa.org       http://www.efa.org

This project focuses on public awareness, consumer and professional education, advocacy, and research on women.

The Brainstorms Companion: Epilepsy in Our View
by Steven C. Schachter
Raven Press
PO Box 1600
Hagerstown, MD 21741
(800) 777-2295                    (301) 714-2300                    FAX (301) 824-7390
http://www.ravenpress.com

In this book, information about epilepsy is presented through the experiences of family members, friends, and associates of people with the condition. Information about types of seizures and living safely with epilepsy is also discussed. $24.00 plus $4.50 shipping and handling.

Brainstorms: Epilepsy in Our Words
by Steven C. Schachter
Raven Press
PO Box 1600
Hagerstown, MD 21741
(800) 777-2295                    (301) 714-2300                    FAX (301) 824-7390
http://www.ravenpress.com

In this book, people with epilepsy describe their seizures and their lives with this condition. Medical information about epilepsy and types of seizures is included. Hardcover, $37.00; softcover, $22.00; plus $4.50 shipping and handling.

Driving: Information for People with Seizure Disorders
Epilepsy Foundation of America (EFA)
4351 Garden City Drive, Suite 406
Landover, MD 20785
(800) 332-1000                    (800) 332-2070 (TT)              (301) 459-3700
FAX (301) 577-2684               (301) 577-0100 (telephone orders only)
e-mail: postmaster@efa.org       http://www.efa.org

This videotape describes how people whose seizures are under control may obtain a driver's license and offers practical advice to those who cannot drive due to uncontrolled seizures. 13 minutes. Available in English and Spanish. Members, $17.96; nonmembers, $19.95.

Epilepsy and the Family
by Richard Lechtenberg
Harvard University Press
79 Garden Street
Cambridge, MA 02138
(800) 448-2242                    (617) 495-2600                    FAX (800) 962-4983
http://www.hup.harvard.edu

In addition to basic information on epilepsy, this book includes chapters on children growing up with a parent who has epilepsy and on siblings and the extended family of individuals with epilepsy. Hardcover, $25.00; softcover, $14.95; plus $3.50 shipping and handling.

Epilepsy A to Z: A Glossary of Epilepsy Terminology
by Peter W. Kaplan, Pierre Loiseau, Robert S. Fisher, and Pierre Jallon
Demos Vermande
386 Park Avenue South, Suite 201
New York, NY 10016
(800) 532-8663                    (212) 683-0072                    FAX (212) 683-0118

This book provides definitions and discussions of terms used in epilepsy including diagnostic procedures and medical and surgical treatments. References to other source materials are also provided. $29.95 plus $4.00 shipping and handling.

Epilepsy: The Untold Stories
by Paul J. Joseph and Mark R. Brown
Fanlight Productions
47 Halifax Street
Boston, MA 02130
(800) 937-4113                    (617) 542-0980                    FAX (617) 542-8838
e-mail: fanlight@tiac.net          http://www.fanlight.com

This videotape, featuring six individuals who have temporal lobe epilepsy, describes how complex partial seizures affect their lives. Also discusses clinical aspects, diagnosis, and treatment of epilepsy. 27 minutes. Purchase, $195.00; rental for one day, $50.00; rental for one week, $100.00; plus $9.00 shipping and handling.

Family Video Library
Epilepsy Foundation of America (EFA)
4351 Garden City Drive, Suite 406
Landover, MD 20785
(800) 332-1000                    (800) 332-2070 (TT)              (301) 459-3700
FAX (301) 577-2684               (301) 577-0100 (telephone orders only)
e-mail: postmaster@efa.org        http://www.efa.org

This collection of videotapes includes subjects such as "Understanding Seizure Disorders," "How Medicines Work," "Epilepsy and the Family," "Living with Epilepsy," "Understanding Complex Partial Seizures," "Epilepsy in the Teen Years," and "The Rest of the Family." Each videotape is $14.95; any four different titles, $48.00; discounts available to members. Many of the videotapes are also available in Spanish. Request "Videos, Books, Guides, & Pamphlets," free.

First Aid for Seizures
Epilepsy Foundation of America (EFA)
4351 Garden City Drive, Suite 406
Landover, MD 20785
(800) 332-1000                    (800) 332-2070 (TT)                    (301) 459-3700
FAX (301) 577-2684               (301) 577-0100 (telephone orders only)
e-mail: postmaster@efa.org       http://www.efa.org

Printed in both English and Spanish, this poster gives simple first aid instruction for people experiencing a seizure. Members, $1.76; nonmembers, $1.95.

A Guide to Understanding and Living with Epilepsy
by Orrin Devinsky
F.A. Davis Company
1915 Arch Street
Philadelphia, PA 19103
(800) 323-3555                    In AK and HI, (215) 440-3001       FAX (215) 440-3016
e-mail: orders@fadavis.com        http://www.fadavis.com

This book discusses medical aspects of epilepsy and its diagnosis and treatment. Also describes epilepsy in children and in adults and legal and financial issues. $15.95

The Legal Rights of Persons with Epilepsy
Epilepsy Foundation of America (EFA)
4351 Garden City Drive, Suite 406
Landover, MD 20785
(800) 332-1000                    (800) 332-2070 (TT)                    (301) 459-3700
FAX (301) 577-2684               (301) 577-0100 (telephone orders only)
e-mail: postmaster@efa.org       http://www.efa.org

This book summarizes legal issues that affect individuals with epilepsy, such as employment, federal benefits, vocational rehabilitation, access to health care, and driving. Members, $13.46; nonmembers, $14.95.

Living Well with Epilepsy
by Robert J. Gumnit
Demos Vermande
386 Park Avenue South, Suite 201
New York, NY 10016
(800) 532-8663                    (212) 683-0072                     FAX (212) 683-0118

Written for health professionals and individuals with epilepsy, this book discusses diagnosis and management of seizure disorders. Hardcover, $19.95; softcover, $13.95; plus $4.00 shipping and handling. $29.95 plus $4.00 shipping and handling.

Management by Common Sense
Epilepsy Foundation of America (EFA)
4351 Garden City Drive, Suite 406
Landover, MD 20785
(800) 332-1000                   (800) 332-2070 (TT)             (301) 459-3700
FAX (301) 577-2684           (301) 577-0100 (telephone orders only)
e-mail: postmaster@efa.org        http://www.efa.org

This booklet, written for employers of individuals with epilepsy, describes the condition and discusses issues such as workers' compensation, effects of medication, and reactions of customers or clients. Members, $1.76; nonmembers, $1.95.

Mother-to-Be: A Guide to Pregnancy and Birth For Women with Disabilities
by Judith Rogers and Molleen Matsumura
Demos Vermande
386 Park Avenue South, Suite 201
New York, NY 10016
(800) 532-8663                   (212) 683-0072              FAX (212) 683-0118

This book describes the pregnancy and childbirth experiences of 36 women with a wide variety of disabilities including epilepsy. Suggests practical solutions for the special concerns of women with disabilities during pregnancy and those of their spouses, families, and health care providers. Includes a list of resources, glossary, and bibliography. $24.95 plus $4.00 shipping and handling.

Parenting and You: A Guide for Parents with Seizure Disorders
When Mom or Dad Has Seizures: A Guide for Young People
Epilepsy Foundation of America (EFA)
4351 Garden City Drive
Landover, MD 20785-2267
(800) 332-1000                   (800) 332-2070 (TT)             (301) 459-3700
FAX (301) 577-2684           (301) 577-0100 (telephone orders only)
e-mail: postmaster@efa.org        http://www.efa.org

"Parenting and You" discusses pregnancy, child care, and parenting issues. "When Mom or Dad Has Seizures" examines how children of various ages might feel about a parent's seizure disorder. Members, $11.66; nonmembers, $12.95 each.

Safety and Seizures: Tips for Living with Seizure Disorders
Epilepsy Foundation of America (EFA)
4351 Garden City Drive, Suite 406
Landover, MD 20785
(800) 332-1000                   (800) 332-2070 (TT)             (301) 459-3700
FAX (301) 577-2684           (301) 577-0100 (telephone orders only)
e-mail: postmaster@efa.org        http://www.efa.org

This brochure provides suggestions for seizure first aid and tips for personal, household, workplace, transportation, parenting, and recreation safety. Members, $.86; nonmembers, $.95.

Seizures and Seniors
Seizures in Later Life
Epilepsy Foundation of America (EFA)
4351 Garden City Drive, Suite 406
Landover, MD 20785
(800) 332-1000                    (800) 332-2070 (TT)              (301) 459-3700
FAX (301) 577-2684               (301) 577-0100 (telephone orders only)
e-mail: postmaster@efa.org       http://www.efa.org

"Seizures and Seniors" provides basic information about epilepsy in older individuals.   Large print.
Members, $.86; nonmembers, $.95.  In the videotape, "Seizures in Later Life," four seniors discuss
the causes of epilepsy and how it affects their lives.  15 minutes.  Members, $17.96; nonmembers,
$19.95.


Voices from the Workplace
Epilepsy Foundation of America (EFA)
4351 Garden City Drive, Suite 406
Landover, MD 20785
(800) 332-1000                    (800) 332-2070 (TT)              (301) 459-3700
FAX (301) 577-2684               (301) 577-0100 (telephone orders only)
e-mail: postmaster@efa.org       http://www.efa.org

Individuals with epilepsy describe the coping strategies they use in the workplace in this videotape.
14 minutes.  Members, $17.96, nonmembers, $19.95.


When the Brain Goes Wrong
Fanlight Productions
47 Halifax Street
Boston, MA 02130
(800) 937-4113                    (617) 542-0980                 FAX (617) 524-8838
e-mail: fanlight@tiac.net        http://www.fanlight.com

This videotape, which deals with seven types of brain dysfunctions, depicts the experiences of an
individual with epilepsy.  45 minutes.  Purchase, $245.00; rental for one day, $50.00; rental for one
week, $100.00; plus $9.00 shipping and handling.


Women and Epilepsy
by Michael R. Trimble (ed.)
John Wiley & Sons
1 Wiley Drive
Somerset, NJ 08875
(800) 225-5945                    (908) 469-4400                 FAX (908) 302-2300

Written by professionals who conduct research, counsel, and treat individuals with epilepsy, this book
focuses on quality of life, reproductive health, pregnancy, sexual functioning, and independent living.
$159.00

<u>The Workbook: A Self-Study Guide for Job-Seekers with Epilepsy</u>
Epilepsy Foundation of America (EFA)
4351 Garden City Drive, Suite 406
Landover, MD 20785
(800) 332-1000                     (800) 332-2070 (TT)                     (301) 459-3700
FAX (301) 577-2684                 (301) 577-0100 (telephone orders only)
e-mail: postmaster@efa.org         http://www.efa.org

This workbook guides individuals with epilepsy in job searches through the use of self-study exercises for finding and retaining employment.  Members, $8.96; nonmembers, $9.95.

# Chapter 7

# *LUPUS*

Being female is the major risk factor for the development of lupus (Hochberg: 1992). Although the exact numbers are not known, various authorities have suggested that lupus affects eight or ten (Arthritis Foundation: 1993) or 10 to 15 (Lahita: 1992) times as many women after puberty as men. The prevalence of lupus among women of childbearing age, mid-teens to mid-40s, is considerably higher than among any other population group. Although the disease may occur in men, children, and elders, it is far less prevalent among these groups. Researchers believe that the immune system is affected by female hormones, thereby putting women at greater risk to develop lupus. Hochberg (1992) reports that incidence, prevalence, and mortality rates for lupus are three times as high in African-American women as in Caucasian women.

Lupus is a chronic disease in which the immune system, which normally protects the body, produces abnormal antibodies that attack the body's connective tissues directly or cause synovitis, an inflammation of the membrane lining the joints (the synovium). The antibodies are produced by the immune system in response to the presence of antigens (foreign materials such as bacteria and viruses) forming antigen-antibody complexes. These "autoantibodies" interfere with blood clotting and cause a variety of symptoms, such as joint swelling and pain, fatigue, skin rashes, pleurisy, and anemia (Lupus Foundation of America: 1993). Lupus autoantibodies may also attack the kidneys, skin, lungs, membranes surrounding the heart, white and red blood cells, and, occasionally, the central nervous system. Lupus and rheumatoid arthritis are considered members of the same family of diseases since both affect the synovium. Nearly half of the individuals who have lupus have arthritis (Fries: 1995).

Diagnosing lupus is difficult, due to the variety of symptoms and their similarity to symptoms of other inflammatory diseases. Its symptoms often occur in flares, when the disease is active, and subside when the disease is in remission. Although there is no cure for lupus, improved diagnostic techniques and medications allow many individuals to continue to live comfortably throughout a normal lifespan.

The cause of lupus is unknown, but scientists suspect that environmental factors such as exposure to ultraviolet rays (sunburn), familial or ethnically determined genetic factors, drug reactions, or hormonal factors, may trigger its symptoms. The National Institute of Arthritis and Musculoskeletal and Skin Diseases has funded two projects that are searching for genetic markers that may be used to identify possible lupus genes. The Lupus Multiplex Registry and Repository in Oklahoma City is enrolling families in which two or more members have been diagnosed with lupus (see "ORGANIZATIONS" section below).

Lupus is diagnosed primarily through patient history, physical exam, and laboratory tests. In addition, urinalysis is used to measure kidney function. Although blood tests may determine the presence of antinuclear antibodies (antibodies that attack cell nuclei) and anti-DNA antibodies (antibodies that attack DNA), often confirming a diagnosis of lupus when other symptoms are present, false positive or false negative results are not uncommon, requiring further monitoring. If diagnosed and treated during the initial acute flare, women with lupus have a good prognosis. It is rare to experience flares after reaching menopause (Berkow: 1987).

## *TYPES OF LUPUS*

*Cutaneous lupus* (or *discoid lupus*) and *systemic lupus erythematosus* (SLE) are the two major types of lupus. A rare condition that is similar to systemic lupus erythematosus may be caused by certain medications used to treat blood pressure or heart problems. This **drug-induced lupus** usually disappears when the medications are discontinued.

**Cutaneous lupus** affects the skin, appearing as red, scaly, raised patches usually found on the face, ears, scalp, arms, and chest. "Butterfly rash" appears most commonly on the cheeks and over the bridge of the nose. The inflammation may be triggered by skin injury or overexposure to sunlight, or it may appear spontaneously with no apparent precipitating cause. Only about ten percent of the individuals who have cutaneous lupus develop the systemic form (Berkow: 1987). Hair loss, scarring, or loss of skin pigmentation may occur. A diagnosis of cutaneous lupus is confirmed by skin biopsy. It is usually treated by topical application or injection of a corticosteroid medication or prescription of an antimalarial drug. To reduce further occurrences of cutaneous lesions, individuals are advised to reduce exposure to sunlight and to use sunscreens with high sun protection factors (SPF). Unlike systemic lupus erythematosus, cutaneous lupus is more common in men than women (Lahita: 1992).

In **systemic lupus erythematosus** (SLE), the immune system malfunctions, producing antibodies that either attack healthy tissues directly or produce an inflammatory reaction, affecting the connective tissues that bind the muscles, joints, and skin together. The manifestations of lupus may vary in the same individual and appear and disappear unpredictably.

In 1982, the American Rheumatism Association (now the American College of Rheumatology) published updated and revised criteria to be considered by physicians when classifying patients with lupus (Tan et al.: 1982). Although the researchers who defined these criteria suggested that they be used mainly in classifying patients, physicians now use these criteria to confirm a diagnosis of systemic lupus erythematosus. If women exhibit four of the 11 criteria, they are considered to have SLE:

- a butterfly shaped rash across cheeks and nose
- discoid rash
- sensitivity to the sun resulting in skin rash
- ulcers or sores in the mouth or nose (usually painless)
- arthritis in two or more joints with swelling or tenderness
- excessive protein in the urine
- inflammation of the tissues around the lung (pleurisy) or heart (pericarditis)
- nervous system disorders such as seizures or psychosis
- immunologic abnormalities revealed through blood tests
- low platelet or white blood cell count or hemolytic anemia
- a positive antinuclear antibody test

About one-third of individuals with SLE develop heart or lung complications (Dibner and Colman: 1994). Heart problems include pericarditis, inflammation of the tissue around the heart; myocarditis, inflammation of the heart muscle; and coronary artery disease, due to high cholesterol levels that are linked to long term treatment with steroids, and high blood pressure, found in women who have kidney problems due to SLE. The lungs may be affected due to inflammation of the lining of the lung.

Some individuals with SLE develop a related condition known as Sjogren's syndrome, which affects the tear, salivary, and other moisture producing glands. Secondary Sjogren's syndrome, in which these symptoms are associated with connective tissue disease, is found in about 10% of individuals with SLE (Wallace: 1995). Corneal erosions, conjunctivitis, and inflammation of the front of the eye are complications of the lack of tears. Sjogren's syndrome is ten times more frequent in women than in men (American College of Rheumatology: no date). Treatment options include artificial tears and ointments or pellets placed between the eyelid and eyeball that dissolve slowly, releasing moisture to the eye. Dry mouth, which may cause swallowing problems and tooth decay, can be relieved by the use of artificial saliva and sugarless gum or candy.

*Lupus nephritis* is one of the most serious complications of SLE. Hughes (no date) believes that "the major factor influencing prognosis is the degree of kidney involvement at the time of diagnosis." Since lupus nephritis is often asymptomatic, urinalysis and blood tests are performed to detect this condition. If ultrasound and kidney biopsy confirm a diagnosis of lupus nephritis, immunosuppressive drugs and corticosteroids are prescribed. If renal failure occurs, dialysis is used to perform kidney function, or a kidney transplant may be performed.

About one-third of all individuals with SLE have antibodies to part of the cell membrane known as the phospholipid. These antiphospholipid antibodies lead to blood clotting abnormalities in about one-third of these individuals (Wallace: 1995). Possible complications caused by antiphospholipid antibodies include miscarriage, stroke, phlebitis (vein inflammation), and pulmonary emboli. Blood tests are used to screen individuals for the presence of antiphospholipid antibodies. Women may be advised to take a baby aspirin daily, or they are treated with an antimalarial drug such as Plaquenil. If a woman has had complications due to a blood clot, anticoagulants such as warfarin (Coumadin) are prescribed.

## TREATMENT FOR LUPUS

Since SLE has varied manifestations and women may experience flares and remission, the medications used to treat it also vary. They include aspirin and other nonsteroidal anti-inflammatory medications (NSAIDS), corticosteroids, and antimalarial drugs. In severe cases, immunosuppressive medications such as cyclophosphamide (Cytoxan) and azathioprine (Imuran) may be prescribed. Each of these medications has potential side effects that must be balanced against benefits. The decision to take these drugs must be made with great caution, obtaining all possible information about the risk factors for experiencing the side effects.

Aspirin relieves the inflammation responsible for joint discomfort and reduces fever but may cause gastrointestinal distress, blood clotting problems, tinnitus (ringing in the ears), and impaired kidney function. Stomach distress may be minimized by choosing coated aspirin or taking the aspirin with milk or a meal. Antacids may be prescribed to counter gastrointestinal discomfort and protect the lining of the stomach. NSAIDS also relieve pain due to inflammation but must be taken with care due to potential gastrointestinal problems, such as diarrhea. The severe side effects of NSAIDS also include the possibility of impaired kidney function and damage to the liver.

Antimalarial drugs such as hydroxychloroquine (Plaquenil) are used to treat the skin rashes of SLE and reduce joint and muscle symptoms, but they also cause digestive system disorders. On rare occasions, the toxicity of antimalarial drugs may cause retinal damage; however, the condition is reversible (Fries: 1995). Women should see an ophthalmologist for an eye examination before treatment with an antimalarial drug and receive follow-up examinations during the course of treatment. Wearing sunglasses with ultra-violet protection and a visor or broad-brimmed hat reduces exposure to sunlight, which may increase the risk of retinal damage (Fries: 1995). Hydroxychloroquine is prescribed most often in the United States, because it is less toxic to the eye.

Corticosteroids (such as prednisone) suppress inflammation dramatically and are often used to treat an active flare, then gradually reduced in periods of remission. "Booster" doses of corticosteroids may be required if the woman is undergoing physical or mental stress. Because corticosteroids cause an increase in appetite, women may experience excessive weight gain that in turn affects weight-bearing joints. Steroids may also hasten the development of osteoporosis, affect diabetes, cause mood swings, and increase blood pressure. The use of steroids should never be stopped abruptly; a gradual reduction under medical supervision is advised. Dehydroepiandrosterone (DHEA), a naturally occurring male hormone, may offer some relief for the side effects of prednisone. Research is currently underway to try to determine if DHEA will diminish lupus flares or improve symptoms when prednisone dosages are reduced (van Vollenhoven: 1996). The Lupus Foundation of America (see "ORGANIZATIONS" section below) can provide information on these trials and enrollment criteria.

Rest, exercise, and diet are also important to women with SLE. During a flare, women often need more rest and should adjust their schedules at home and at work. Alternating rest and activity periods may help the individual maintain as close to normal a schedule as possible. When a flare subsides, it is important to exercise in order to avoid muscle weakness and joint stiffness. A physical therapist can design an exercise program, taking the individual's physical capacity and daily schedule into account. Exercise may also help women feel more fit and better about themselves.

## SEXUAL FUNCTIONING

When SLE makes activities of daily living difficult, it may affect interpersonal relationships. These problems combined with mood changes due to medication and the need for the woman's partner to take on some of the roles she normally takes may also lead to sexual problems (Gerber: 1988). The woman with SLE may lose her sense of self-esteem, becoming self-conscious about body-image due to weight gain associated with use of steroid drugs; skin rash; hair loss; and lack of energy. Regular exercise may help reduce weakness, contribute to weight control, and increase feelings of well-being.

Medications taken to reduce pain may also reduce libido. A woman may also fear pain during intimacy, while her partner may fear causing pain. Vaginal dryness may be reduced through the use of a commercial, water soluble lubricant. Fatigue and a diminished range of motion may also affect sexual function. Anti-inflammatory medication should be scheduled so that it will provide maximum relief during sexual relations without reducing arousal. A warm bath or shower may help to relax joints and muscles. Changing positions for intercourse may also reduce joint pain and improve sexual relations.

Communication between partners is key to living with a chronic disease as well as to maintaining sexual function. Relationships that were weak prior to the onset of SLE may be threatened by the adjustments needed in everyday life. Both partners may benefit from counseling.

## FAMILY PLANNING, PREGNANCY, AND CHILDREARING

Couples must weigh the decision to have children carefully, as the flares of SLE usually occur during childbearing years. They must evaluate the risk to both mother and fetus, the effects of treatment for autoantibodies, and the effects on the family. Medications may affect fertility in the woman experiencing a flare. It is a good idea to seek obstetric care from a physician who not only has experience in the management of high risk pregnancies, but who is also willing to work with the rheumatologist to provide the best possible care.

Women who do not wish to become pregnant are advised to choose contraceptive methods with care. Women who have the antiphospholipid syndrome or other blood clotting problems, migraine headaches, high blood pressure, or a high cholesterol level are advised not to take birth control pills containing estrogen, due to an increased risk for stroke or other conditions caused by blood clots (Wallace: 1995). Diaphragms, used with contraceptive foam or gel, and condoms are better choices.

Couples should also consider the potential for stress on the partner due to the extra duties necessitated by pregnancy fatigue; concerns about passing on the disease to offspring; and the emotional stress caused by a greater chance of miscarriage due to abnormal antibodies in the mother's blood. Financial matters may be an issue if the couple is dependent on the wife's earnings. The physical tasks of baby care, such as lifting, bathing, and carrying the infant, must be planned in advance in the event the disease flares after delivery. Other children in the family, born before the mother was diagnosed with SLE, may need special attention to cope with the mother's new disabilities as well as a new sibling.

Hayslett (1992), in an analysis of the effects of SLE on pregnancy and pregnancy outcomes, reported that the best outcomes were experienced by women who were in remission at pregnancy onset. Pregnancy should be considered carefully in women with poor kidney function, since both mother and fetus may be affected (Rogers and Matsumura: 1991). A woman with lupus nephritis is more likely to have a flare during pregnancy. Immunosuppressive drugs should be discontinued before conception, but the use of steroids does not cause birth defects. Aspirin may help reduce the risk of toxemia of pregnancy (preeclampsia), a combination of increased blood pressure and protein in the urine that poses risks for both mother and baby. Hughes (no date) reports that although there is no increased risk of flares during pregnancy, the risk of flares increases after delivery. These flares are usually mild. Some physicians prescribe a steroid injection ten days to two weeks postpartum to avoid flares (Wallace: 1995).

The potential risks to the fetus include a greater than average risk of prematurity, retarded growth, and death. In the first trimester, there is a greater risk of fetal death due to placental damage (blood clotting) resulting in miscarriage. Ferris and Reece (1994) report rates of fetal loss of 5 to 15% in women with inactive SLE; 20 to 50% in women with active disease. Antibodies that interfere with the placenta are found in about a third of the women with SLE. Blood tests should be performed to determine the presence of these antibodies, since their presence indicates a high risk for fetal loss (Julkunen et al.: 1993). Blood clots may form in the placenta, interfering with fetal nourishment and retarding fetal growth (Lockshin: 1992).

Problems later in pregnancy may be caused by kidney failure or high blood pressure in the mother. Ultrasound should be used to determine gestational age in order to determine whether there is growth retardation or risk of premature birth. There is also the risk of premature labor. Cesarean delivery is more common in mothers with SLE, due to prematurity or fetal distress. Transient skin rashes or low blood counts may be symptomatic of neonatal lupus; the only congenital defect resulting from maternal lupus is a slow heart rate. Steroid drug dosage is often increased prior to delivery but decreased subsequently, since steroids may interfere with breast milk production. Mothers may be advised not to breastfeed, since antimalarial and immunosuppressive drugs are passed through breast milk to the baby.

## *PSYCHOLOGICAL ASPECTS OF LUPUS*

Women with chronic diseases such as SLE experience a wide range of emotions, such as depression, loss of self-esteem, and worry, which in turn make everyday life even more difficult. Denial, anger, and depression are classic responses, eventually leading to resolution. In rheumatic diseases such as SLE, this grieving cycle may be repeated as flares and remissions occur throughout the disease course (Partridge: 1988). Pain and fatigue are major manifestations of SLE, causing women to mourn the loss of their previous good health. They may find it difficult to learn how to adjust to the flares and remissions; to cope with the pain and possible changes in their appearance; and to undergo a medical treatment program. About half of all individuals with SLE develop neurological problems such as central nervous system disease and clinical depression. In some women, treatment with high dose of corticosteroids may lead to psychological distress and impaired cognitive functioning (Iverson: 1995).

It is important for the physician to explain these aspects of this chronic disease to the woman and her family and to suggest coping strategies. Family members must try to understand that symptoms may vary day-to-day. Overwhelming fatigue may occur without warning or outward symptoms, forcing changes in schedules. It may be necessary for family members to shoulder additional responsibilities in the home or to obtain household help. At times family members may be overprotective; at other times, they may want to disassociate themselves from the woman with SLE, resisting change and refusing to acknowledge her illness. It is crucial for the family and the woman with SLE to discuss their feelings of frustration, impatience, and resentment. Women with SLE must learn to ask for help rather than suffer in silence, while family members must become comfortable enough to suggest alternatives to old routines.

Strategies that may help the woman with SLE to continue working include education and environmental adaptations. She should explain the flares associated with SLE and how they may affect her work to her employer and ask about the possibility of a flexible schedule. Employees with SLE should avoid offices with windows and skylights to minimize sunlight exposure. It is also important to maintain a constant temperature in the office. If a job is physically demanding, it may be wise to consider a change.

The Arthritis Foundation recommends learning stress reduction or relaxation techniques and participating in recreational activities and social groups. A seven week Systemic Lupus Erythematosus Self-Help Course is offered by many local chapters of the Arthritis Foundation. The Lupus Foundation of America also serves individuals, their families, and health professionals (see "ORGANIZATIONS" section below).

## PROFESSIONAL SERVICE PROVIDERS

*Rheumatologists* are physicians who specialize in the diagnosis and treatment of rheumatic diseases, which are inflammations and degenerations of connective tissues and joints. *Dermatologists* are physicians who specialize in the diagnosis and treatment of skin problems. Dermatologists may perform skin biopsies to confirm a diagnosis of cutaneous lupus. *Obstetricians* are physicians who provide primary care during pregnancy, labor and delivery, and postpartum. Some may be specialists in treating women with high risk pregnancies due to chronic disease; they should work with the woman's rheumatologist to provide multidisciplinary care during pregnancy.

*Occupational therapists* teach women with SLE new techniques to perform everyday activities, such as washing and dressing, homemaking, and recreation. Many assistive devices, such as reaching tools, built-up kitchen utensils, and writing aids, may be suggested.

*Physical therapists* design exercise programs with strengthening and range of motion exercises to keep women with SLE moving as easily as possible despite flares with joint pain and fatigue.

*Social workers* provide information about financial and medical benefits, housing, and community resources. They conduct individual, family, or group counseling and may refer individuals to self-help or peer counseling groups.

*Rehabilitation counselors* help individuals with lupus develop a plan that will enable them to continue functioning and working. Some individuals will need assistance in returning to their previous position or retraining to obtain a different type of position. Rehabilitation counselors help make the contacts and placements necessary to attain these goals.

The health care professionals who provide services to women with SLE work in hospitals, rehabilitation centers, home health agencies, private and public agencies, independent living centers, and as private practitioners. Individual and group counseling may be available through a local hospital, community health center, or from mental health professionals in private practice. Members of self-help groups, often run under the auspices of voluntary associations, share emotional support and practical advice. Some women attend pain clinics which teach behavior modification techniques to limit the effect of pain.

Women who are severely disabled by SLE often require home health services. These services are provided by nurses or home health agencies; special homemaker services; Meals on Wheels programs; chore services such as housecleaning; and adult day activity programs. The services are often free to women with low income, or fees may be charged on a sliding scale.

The desire to remain independent provides strong motivation for rehabilitation. Patient education programs offered by hospitals, universities, and health organization chapters teach self-management skills to women with SLE in order to help them live as independently as possible. These courses often result in reduction in pain, dependency, and depression (National Resource Center on Health Promotion and Aging: 1989). Common topics in these courses are education about SLE, emotional support, and discussions of how women can advocate for themselves within the health care system and participate in choosing treatment options. Many women with SLE experience problems in obtaining or retaining medical insurance. Social Security Disability Insurance (SSDI) is often denied due to the patterns of flares and remissions. Group members, patient advocates in hospitals, and participants in courses can relate their experiences and offer strategies that have been effective in appealing these denials.

References

American College of Rheumatology
No date Fact Sheet: Sjogren's Syndrome Atlanta, GA: American College of Rheumatology
Arthritis Foundation
1993 Systemic Lupus Erythematosus Atlanta, GA: Arthritis Foundation
Berkow, Robert
1987 "Discoid Lupus Erythematosus" pp. 1273-1274 in Robert Berkow (ed.) The Merck Manual of Diagnosis and Therapy Rahway, NJ: Merck & Co.
Dibner, Robin and Carol Colman
1994 The Lupus Handbook for Women New York, NY: Simon & Schuster
Ferris, Ann M. and E. Albert Reece
1994 "Nutritional Consequences of Chronic Maternal Conditions During Pregnancy and Lactation: Lupus and Diabetes" American Journal of Clinical Nutrition 59:February:2 Supplement:465S-4673S
Fries, James F.
1995 Arthritis: A Take Care of Yourself Health Guide Reading, MA: Addison-Wesley Publishing Company
Gerber, Lynn H.
1988 "Rehabilitative Therapies for Patients with Rheumatic Disease" pp. 301-307 in H. Ralph Schumacher, Jr. (ed.) Primer on the Rheumatic Diseases Atlanta, GA: Arthritis Foundation

Hayslett, J.P.
1992 "The Effect of Systemic Lupus Erythematosus on Pregnancy and Pregnancy Outcome" American Journal of Reproductive Immunology 28(3-4):199-204

Hochberg, Marc D.
1992 "Epidemiology of Systemic Lupus Erythematosus" pp. 103-117 in Robert C. Lahita (ed.) Systemic Lupus Erythematosus New York, NY: Churchill Livingstone

Hughes, Graham R.V.
No date Lupus: A Guide for Patients Torrance, CA: American Lupus Society

Iverson, Grant L.
1995 "The Need for Psychological Services for Persons with Systemic Lupus Erythematosus" Rehabilitation Psychology 40:1:39-49

Julkunen, H. et al.
1993 "Fetal Outcome in Lupus Pregnancy: A Retrospective Case-Control of 242 Pregnancies in 112 Patients" Lupus April:2(2):125-31

Lahita, Robert G.
1992 "The Early Diagnosis of Systemic Lupus Erythematosus" Journal of Women's Health 1:2:117-121
1992 Lupus in Men Rockville, MD: Lupus Foundation of America

Lockshin, Michael D.
1992 Pregnancy and Lupus Rockville, MD: Lupus Foundation of America

Lupus Foundation of America
1993 Lupus Rockville, MD: Lupus Foundation of America

National Resource Center on Health Promotion and Aging
1989 "Arthritis: Positive Approaches Offer New Hope" Perspectives in Health Promotion and Aging 4:(November-December)6

Partridge, Alison J.
1988 "Psychosocial Aspects of the Rheumatic Diseases" pp. 307-309 in H. Ralph Schumacher, Jr. (ed.) Primer on the Rheumatic Diseases Atlanta, GA: Arthritis Foundation

Rogers, Judith and Molleen Matsumura
1991 Mother-to-Be: A Guide to Pregnancy and Birth for Women with Disabilities New York, NY: Demos Publications

Tan, Eng M. et al.
1982 "The 1982 Revised Criteria for the Classification of Systemic Lupus Erythematosus" Arthritis and Rheumatism 25(November 1982):11:1271-77

van Vollenhoven, Ron
1996 "Update on DHEA Research at Stanford University" Bay Area Lupus Foundation Newsletter 19:4:5

Wallace, Daniel J.
1995 The Lupus Book: A Guide for Patients and Their Families New York, NY: Oxford University Press

# ORGANIZATIONS

American College of Rheumatology
60 Executive Park South, Suite 150
Atlanta, GA 30329
(404) 633-3777                    FAX (404) 633-1870
http://www.rheumatology.org

A professional membership organization for rheumatologists who treat or study all forms of arthritis and associated diseases such as lupus. Will provide a state-by-state list of rheumatologists.

Arthritis Foundation
1314 Spring Street, NW
Atlanta, GA 30309
(800) 283-7800              (404) 872-7100              FAX (404) 872-0457
http://www@arthritis.org

Supports research in rheumatic diseases, including lupus; offers referrals to rheumatologists; provides public and professional education; sponsors classes and clubs; and offers discount drug services. Chapters and divisions across the U.S. Membership, $20.00, includes chapter newsletter and bimonthly magazine, "Arthritis Today."

Arthritis Society
250 Bloor Street East, Suite 401
Toronto, Ontario M4W 3P2 Canada
(416) 967-1414              FAX (416) 967-7171
http://www.arthritis.ca

Supports research on the causes and cures for lupus and other rheumatic diseases; sponsors medical training programs; provides information and educational materials; establishes self-help groups; and in some provinces, offers home-visit programs. Division offices in every province. Publishes "Arthritis News" and "Communique" (in French), quarterly. Subscription, $10.00.

L.E. Support Club
8039 Nova Court
North Charleston, SC 29420-8934
(803) 764-1769

Provides educational and emotional support to members. Provides Patient Medication Instruction Sheets which describe individual medications, instructions for use, precautions, and side effects. Membership, U.S., $20.00 (bulk rate postage) or $23.00 (first class postage); Canada, $22.00; includes bimonthly newsletter, "L.E. Beacon."

**Lupus Foundation of America**
1300 Piccard Drive, Suite 200
Rockville, MD 20850-4303
(301) 670-9292                    (800) 558-0121 (Recorded Information Tape Line only)
http://www.lupus.org/lupus

Supports lupus research, provides public education about lupus, and assists more than 90 local chapters in serving individuals with lupus and their families. Publishes quarterly newsletter, "Lupus News," $20.00.

**Lupus Multiplex Registry and Repository**
Oklahoma Medical Research Foundation
825 Northeast 13th Street
Oklahoma City, OK 73104
(800) 522-0211, ext. 7479           (405) 271-3046           FAX (405) 271-3045
http://omrf.uokhsc.edu/lupus

Sponsored by the National Institute of Arthritis, Musculoskeletal and Skin Diseases, this center conducts genetic studies of families that have at least two members diagnosed with lupus. Currently recruiting study participants. Requires blood sample and medical history interview. Publishes annual newsletter, "The Lupus Linkage Newsletter," free.

**Lupus Network**
230 Ranch Drive
Bridgeport, CT 06606
(203) 372-5795

Provides information about lupus through medical briefs, personal stories, book reviews, and articles about coping with lupus. Membership, U.S., $10.00; Canada, $13.00; includes quarterly newsletter, "Heliogram."

**National Arthritis and Musculoskeletal and Skin Diseases Information Clearinghouse**
1 AMS Circle
Bethesda, MD 20892
(301) 495-4484                    (301) 565-2966 (TT)           FAX (301) 587-4352

Compiles and distributes information to health care professionals. Distributes bibliographies, fact sheets, catalogues, and directories. Requests from consumers are referred to the Arthritis Foundation.

**National Institute of Arthritis and Musculoskeletal and Skin Diseases** (NIAMS)
Building 31, Room 4C-32
9000 Rockville Pike
Bethesda, MD 20892
(301) 496-8190                    FAX (301) 480-6069           http://www.nih.gov/niams

Sponsors Multi-Purpose Arthritis Centers, which conduct basic and clinical research; provide professional, public, and patient education; and sponsor community activities and educational programs, including the Task Force on Lupus in High Risk Populations, directed to African-American women who are at greater risk for lupus than Caucasian women. Distributes a program planning kit, "What Black Women Should Know About Lupus: Ideas for Community Programs," free.

National Sjogren's Syndrome Association
PO Box 42207
Phoenix, AZ 85080-2207
(800) 395-6772                    (602) 516-0787                    FAX (602) 516-0111
e-mail: NSSA@aol.com

Provides information to individuals and professionals through support groups and conferences throughout the U.S.  Membership, $25.00, includes quarterly "Patient Education Series" and newsletter, "Sjogren's Digest."

Sjogren's Syndrome Foundation
333 North Broadway
Jericho, NY 11753
(800) 475-6473                    (516) 933-6365                    FAX (516) 933-6368
http://www.w2.com/ss.html

Provides information to individuals and professionals through support groups and conferences throughout the U.S., Canada, and abroad.  Membership, U.S., $25.00; Canada, $30.00;  includes bimonthly newsletter, "The Moisture Seekers."

Arthritis and Everyday Living
Therapy Skill Builders
555 Academic Court
San Antonio, TX 78204-2498
(800) 228-0752                    (800) 723-1318 (TT)                    FAX (800) 232-1223
e-mail: customer_service@hbtpc.com

This instructional videotape demonstrates techniques for everyday household activities and shows assistive devices. 30 minutes. Viewer's guide included. $65.00 plus 10% shipping and handling.

Arthritis and Pregnancy
Arthritis Foundation
1314 Spring Street, NW
Atlanta, GA 30309
(800) 283-7800                    (404) 872-7100                    FAX (404) 872-0457
http://www@arthritis.org

This booklet provides information for women with lupus, as well as other forms of arthritis. Discusses how pregnancy affects lupus and vice versa. Includes a self-test for strength and endurance and suggestions for saving energy and protecting joints when caring for a baby. Free

Arthritis: A Take Care of Yourself Health Guide
by James F. Fries
Addison-Wesley-Longman Publishing Company
1 Jacob Way
Reading, MA 01867
(800) 447-2226                    (617) 944-3700

This book describes the major forms of arthritis, including lupus, and methods of managing the condition through exercise, medication, or surgery. Suggests problem solving techniques for pain, mobility, sexual function, and employment. $14.00

Arthritis, Rheumatic Diseases, and Related Disorders
National Arthritis and Musculoskeletal and Skin Diseases Information Clearinghouse
1 AMS Circle
Bethesda, MD 20892
(301) 495-4484                    (301) 565-2966 (TT)                    FAX (301) 587-4352

This 1993 Special Report provides highlights of the research activities sponsored by the National Institutes of Health, including research on lupus. Free

Aspirin and Other NSAID's
Arthritis Foundation
1314 Spring Street, NW
Atlanta, GA 30309
(800) 283-7800          (404) 872-7100          FAX (404) 872-0457
http://www@arthritis.org

Using a question and answer format, this booklet discusses NSAIDs and possible side effects.  Free

Coping with Lupus
by Robert H. Phillips
Avery Publishing Group
120 Old Broadway
Garden City Park, NY 11040
(800) 548-5757          (516) 741-2155          FAX (516) 742-1892

Written by a psychologist, this book provides information for everyday living with lupus for individuals with the condition and their families.  $12.95 plus $3.00 shipping and handling.

Facts About Lupus
Lupus Foundation of America
1300 Piccard Drive, Suite 200
Rockville, MD 20850-4303
(301) 670-9292          (800) 558-0121 (Recorded Information Tape Line only)
http://www.lupus.org/lupus

This series of brochures discusses lupus symptoms, diagnostic tests, medications, and suggestions for coping with this chronic condition.  $3.95

Living and Loving: Information About Sex
Arthritis Foundation
1314 Spring Street, NW
Atlanta, GA 30309
(800) 283-7800          (404) 872-7100          FAX (404) 872-0457
http://www@arthritis.org

This booklet discusses the effects that medication, physical problems, and emotional responses may have on sexuality in individuals with rheumatic diseases, including lupus, and their partners.  It also makes suggestions for improving sexual relations.  Free

Living with Lupus
by Sheldon Paul Blau with Dodi Schultz
Addison-Wesley-Longman Publishing Company
1 Jacob Way
Reading, MA 01867
(800) 447-2226          (617) 944-3700

This book discusses many aspects of lupus, including diagnostic techniques, treatment, patient-physician relationships, and current research. Includes a glossary and bibliography. $12.00

Living with Lupus: A Comprehensive Guide to Understanding and Controlling Lupus While Getting On With Your Life
by Mark Horowitz and Marietta Abrams Brill
Penguin USA
120 Woodbine Street
Bergenfield, NJ 07621
(800) 253-6476

Co-authored by a rheumatologist, this book provides guidelines for understanding and coping with lupus. Includes a chapter on pregnancy and parenthood. $11.95 plus $2.00 shipping and handling.

Lupus
Arthritis Foundation
1314 Spring Street, NW
Atlanta, GA 30309
(800) 283-7800                    (404) 872-7100                    FAX (404) 872-0457
http://www@arthritis.org

This booklet describes diagnosis and treatment of lupus and its relation to pregnancy and contraception; it also suggests coping strategies. Free

Lupus
National Arthritis and Musculoskeletal and Skin Diseases Information Clearinghouse
1 AMS Circle
Bethesda, MD 20892
(301) 495-4484                    (301) 565-2966 (TT)                    FAX (301) 587-4352

This information packet contains medical articles, patient information, fact sheets, and a glossary. Also lists Multi-Purpose Arthritis Centers where lupus research is conducted. Free

The Lupus Book: A Guide for Patients and Their Families
by Daniel J. Wallace
Oxford University Press
2001 Evans Road
Cary, NC 27513
(800) 451-7556                    FAX (919) 677-1303
e-mail: orders@oup-usa.org       http://www.oup-usa.org

Written by a rheumatologist, this book describes the diagnosis and treatment of lupus. Includes discussions of the immune system and descriptions of the effects of the condition on other bodily systems. $25.00

The Lupus Handbook for Women
by Robin Dibner and Carol Colman
Simon and Schuster
200 Old Tappan Road
Old Tappan, NJ 07675
(800) 223-2348                    e-mail: ss cust serv@prenhall.com
http://www.simonsays.com

Co-authored by a rheumatologist, this book provides information about diagnosis and treatment with an emphasis on self-management, relationships, pregnancy, and parenting. $11.00 plus $3.00 shipping and handling.

Lupus: Living with It: Why You Don't Have to Be Healthy to Be Happy
by Suzy Szasz
Prometheus Books
59 John Glenn Drive
Amherst, NY 14228-2197
(800) 421-0351                    FAX (716) 691-0137
e-mail: pbooks6205@aol.com        http://www.prometheusbooks.com

Written by a woman who has lupus, this book describes her experiences from adolescence to adulthood in dealing with lupus flares, hospitalizations, and treatment, while pursuing an education and a professional career. $16.95 plus $4.45 shipping and handling.

Lupus: My Search for a Diagnosis
by Eileen Radziunas
Hunter House
PO Box 2914
Alameda, CA 94501-0914
(800) 266-5592              (510) 865-5282              FAX (510) 865-4295
http://www.hunterhouse.com

This book provides the personal account of the author's struggle to find a diagnosis, including her frustrations resulting from the lack of understanding in the medical community. Describes the effects of an unknown chronic disease on family relationships and friends. Discusses the need for a case management approach by health care professionals. $8.95 plus $4.50 shipping and handling.

Mother-to-Be: A Guide to Pregnancy and Birth For Women with Disabilities
by Judith Rogers and Molleen Matsumura
Demos Vermande
386 Park Avenue South, Suite 201
New York, NY 10016
(800) 532-8663              (212) 683-0072              FAX (212) 683-0118

This book describes the pregnancy and childbirth experiences of 36 women with a wide variety of disabilities including systemic lupus erythematosus. Suggests practical solutions for the special concerns of individuals with disabilities during pregnancy and those of their partners, families, and health care providers. Includes a list of resources, glossary, and bibliography. $24.95 plus $4.00 shipping and handling.

Sjogren's Syndrome
Arthritis Foundation
1314 Spring Street, NW
Atlanta, GA 30309
(800) 283-7800          (404) 872-7100          FAX (404) 872-0457
http://www@arthritis.org

This booklet explains the causes, symptoms, diagnosis, and treatment for this related condition. Free

The Sjogren's Syndrome Handbook
Sjogren's Syndrome Foundation
333 North Broadway
Jericho, NY 11753
(800) 475-6473          (516) 933-6365          FAX (516) 933-6368
http://www.w2.com/ss.html

This book provides practical suggestions for living more comfortably with this chronic condition. Members, $19.95; nonmembers, $29.95; plus $2.50 shipping and handling; shipping to Canada, $7.00.

We Are Not Alone: Learning to Live with Chronic Illness
by Sefra Kobrin Pitzele
Workman Publishing
708 Broadway
New York, NY 10003
(800) 722-7202          (212) 254-5900

Written by a woman with lupus, this book offers practical advice for coping with chronic diseases and maintaining relationships. It also provides practical suggestions for independent living. $10.95 plus $3.00 shipping and handling.

What Black Women Should Know About Lupus
National Arthritis and Musculoskeletal and Skin Diseases Clearinghouse
1 AMS Circle
Bethesda, MD 20892
(301) 495-4484          (301) 565-2966 (TT)          FAX (301) 587-4352

This pamphlet describes types, symptoms, and treatment of lupus. Available in large print, braille, and audiocassette. Free

<u>When Mom Gets Sick</u>
by Rebecca Samuels
Lupus Foundation of America
1300 Piccard Drive, Suite 200
Rockville, MD 20850-4303
(301) 670-9292                     (800) 558-0121 (Recorded Information Tape Line only)
http://www.lupus.org/lupus

This book was written by a young girl whose mother has lupus.  $6.95 plus $4.50 shipping and handling.

# Chapter 8

# MULTIPLE SCLEROSIS

Multiple sclerosis (MS) is a chronic central nervous system condition in which the nerve fibers of the brain and spinal cord are damaged. A fatty substance called myelin protects the nerve fibers and enables the smooth transmission of neurological impulses between the central nervous system and the rest of the body. If inflammation damages or destroys the myelin, it may heal with no loss of function. Later, however, scar (or plaque) may form and interfere with the transmission of neurological impulses. Function may be diminished or lost. The disease is called multiple sclerosis because there are multiple areas of scarring or sclerosis (Minden and Frankel: 1989).

Multiple sclerosis affects twice as many women as men and twice as many whites as African-Americans (Scheinberg and Smith: 1989). Age of onset ranges from mid to late adolescence to middle age. Estimates of the number of individuals with multiple sclerosis vary from less than 200,000, based on hospital and physicians' records, to 500,000, based on public surveys and pathology records (National Institute of Neurological Disorders and Stroke: 1990).

Nearly 77% of individuals with multiple sclerosis have activity limitations (National Center for Health Statistics: 1988). The broad economic and social implications of multiple sclerosis include medical expenses, unemployment or underemployment, the cost of special services, and the emotional and physical effects on the individual and family members. Cognitive problems such as memory loss, forgetfulness, and the inability to maintain a train of thought have been reported by many individuals with multiple sclerosis (Sullivan et al.: 1990).

Each woman with multiple sclerosis has unique symptoms based on the location of the damage to the nervous system. These symptoms may include blurred or double vision, numbness in the extremities, balance or coordination problems, fatigue, muscle spasticity or stiffness, slurred speech, muscle weakness, or loss of bladder or bowel control.

The cause of multiple sclerosis is unknown. Scientists who believe that multiple sclerosis is an autoimmune disease are investigating the role of a variety of viruses in triggering damage to the immune system, which in turn may lead to the development of multiple sclerosis. Other investigators are studying the role of heredity. Their studies suggest that certain genetic factors may predispose some individuals to acquire multiple sclerosis, but there is no known pattern of direct inheritance.

## DIAGNOSIS OF MULTIPLE SCLEROSIS

A diagnosis of multiple sclerosis is made if there is evidence of two episodes of functional loss at least a month apart; clinical evidence of at least one lesion; and another separate lesion confirmed by laboratory evidence (Calvano: 1991). The development of magnetic resonance imaging (MRI), which provides a recorded image of central nervous system lesions, has led to improved diagnostic techniques for multiple sclerosis. The MRIs images are produced by the interaction between its magnetic field and the hydrogen atoms in body cells. The MRI is considered to be nearly 90% accurate in diagnosing multiple sclerosis (Calvano: 1989). Because MRIs are so accurate, diagnostic procedures used in the past, such as CT scans (which use x-rays to scan the central nervous system for signs of demyelination), lumbar punctures, and myelography (an x-ray procedure), are now used infrequently.

Evoked potentials (EP) studies measure how fast electrical impulses travel through the central nervous system to the brain and are used in conjunction with the MRI. The physician may use one of three evoked potentials to assess various losses of function. The visual evoked potential assesses the visual pathway to the optic nerve; the somatosensory evoked potential studies sensory reactions and limb and spinal cord nerve function; and the brainstem auditory evoked potential may reveal the cause of hearing and balance problems. Evoked potentials are performed on an outpatient basis. Electrodes are placed on the skin, using a conducting ointment. A mild electrical stimulus is administered by the technician, and a computer records the brain's response to the stimulus. The physician studies the computer recordings to determine the site of neurological damage.

## TYPES OF MULTIPLE SCLEROSIS

In 1996, an international panel of physicians who treat individuals with multiple sclerosis recommended that the following terms be used to describe the types of multiple sclerosis (Reingold: 1996). *Relapsing-remitting* describes a pattern of multiple sclerosis in which exacerbations are followed by either full recovery or partial recovery and lasting disability. Individuals with the *primary progressive* form experience steady disease progression. The *secondary progressive* form has a clear pattern of relapses and recovery, becoming progressively worse between acute exacerbations. *Progressive-relapsing* multiple sclerosis is progressive from onset with acute attacks.

These forms of multiple sclerosis are not exclusive; some individuals may experience progression from one form to another. Smith and Scheinberg (1985) report that there is a more favorable prognosis for individuals with early onset (before age 35); acute onset rather than gradual onset; complete remission after the first attack; and sensory rather than motor symptoms.

## TREATMENT OF MULTIPLE SCLEROSIS

There is no cure for multiple sclerosis; however, physicians can treat the symptoms of multiple sclerosis and try to control its progress with anti-inflammatory medication.

In 1993, the Food and Drug Administration (FDA) gave its approval for the use of interferon beta-1b (Betaseron) in treating ambulatory individuals ages 18 to 50 with relapsing-remitting multiple sclerosis. Clinical studies have shown that Betaseron reduces the frequency and severity of exacerbations. MRI studies have shown a reduced number and size of brain lesions after using Betaseron (Goodkin: 1995). Betaseron is injected by the individual subcutaneously every other day. The most common side effects reported are reactions at the injection site, such as swelling, redness, rashes, and flu-like symptoms, including chills, fatigue, fever, and muscle aches. Individuals using Betaseron must learn to inject the drug and determine an injection schedule that works best for them, minimizing side effects. Betaseron is expensive, nearly $10,000 per year. The Betaseron Foundation aids underinsured individuals to obtain the medication.

Interferon beta-1a (Avonex) has been shown to reduce disease activity in individuals with relapsing-remitting multiple sclerosis and to slow the progression of disability. Avonex is administered in a once-a-week intramuscular injection into the thigh, hip, or upper arm. Many individuals self-inject or receive treatments from a caregiver. In clinical trials, the major side effect was initial flu-like symptoms which diminished over the course of treatment. Women who are pregnant or who are trying to become pregnant should not use Avonex. Biogen, the manufacturer of Avonex, offers a toll-free support line and literature to individuals (see "ORGANIZATIONS section below).

Copolymer I (Copaxone) was recommended for approval in September, 1996 by an FDA advisory panel and is awaiting additional review. Copaxone may potentially reduce relapse rates in individuals with relapsing-remitting multiple sclerosis (National Multiple Sclerosis Society: 1995). It is injected subcutaneously on a daily basis. Teva Marion Partners, the manufacturer of Copaxone has developed a customized patient support program called "Shared Solutions" (see "ORGANIZ-ATIONS" section below).

Prednisone, adrenocorticotropic hormone (ACTH), prednisolone, and other anti-inflammatory drugs have been effective in reducing the severity and duration of multiple sclerosis flare-ups. These medications are not recommended for long term use because of side effects such as nausea, drowsiness, changes in blood pressure and blood glucose levels, lowered resistance to infection, and thinning of bones (Lechtenberg: 1995). Medication may also be used to treat multiple sclerosis symptoms such as spasticity, dizziness, fatigue, bladder problems, tremors, depression, and sensory problems (a "pins and needles" feeling). The woman with multiple sclerosis and the physician must carefully consider each medication and its possible side effects, which may appear to be symptoms of the disease itself.

*Optic neuritis*, *double vision*, and *nystagmus* are common visual symptoms of multiple sclerosis. Inflammation of the optic nerve (neuritis) causes loss of vision. If the muscles of the eye are weakened by nerve demyelination, the woman cannot focus and experiences double vision (diplopia). Double vision may occur during an exacerbation and disappear during remission of multiple sclerosis symptoms. Cortisone is often used to treat optic neuritis and double vision. Nystagmus is an involuntary rapid eye movement; it interferes with focusing and may cause dizziness.

Some women with multiple sclerosis experience *problems with gait* including weakness, spasticity, and lack of coordination (ataxia). Antispastic medications, stretching exercises, and swimming may relieve the symptoms of stiff gait, foot drop, and toe dragging. Orthoses are assistive devices used to support weakened areas, provide proper alignment, and improve function. An ankle foot orthosis worn inside the shoe may relieve the symptoms of spasticity. Ataxia is treated with a sequential exercise program in which the individual performs repetitive movements, often watching herself in a mirror, to increase sensory feedback and restore coordination.

About 80% of individuals with multiple sclerosis experience *urinary dysfunction* (Holland: 1996). Urinary tract infections, formation of bladder stones, and kidney damage may occur if the bladder is not completely emptied during voiding. Symptoms of urinary dysfunction include urgency, frequency, hesitancy, nocturia (waking up to urinate during the night), and incontinence. Symptoms of urinary tract infections may include discomfort when urinating, frequent urination, fever, and urine that smells unpleasant. Antibiotics are used to treat urinary tract infections. To avoid further problems, women, who are at greater risk for these infections (Schapiro: 1994), are advised to empty their bladders completely; wear cotton undergarments; drink six to eight glasses of fluid per day; take vitamin C; practice careful personal hygiene, wiping from front to back after voiding or bowel movements; and, for those who use catheters, keeping equipment clean. Although some women with occasional incontinence rely on absorbent undergarments, medications and catheterization are used when symptoms are more severe. Anticholinergic drugs may be used to control bladder dysfunction by regulating bladder contractions (Lechtenberg: 1995). In intermittent self-catheterization, a flexible catheter is inserted through the urethra into the bladder at planned intervals in order to empty it. Many individuals find that self-catheterization allows the bladder to regain normal function. (Holland: 1996).

*Constipation* is the most common bowel problem and may be caused by inadequate fluid and fiber consumption, medication, lack of physical activity, and decreased sensation in the rectal area. Eating high fiber foods, drinking eight to 12 cups of liquid daily, increasing physical activity, and using stool softeners or bulk formers (if necessary), are important in a bowel management program that will reduce symptoms and discomfort. To avoid constipation, women should develop a regular schedule for bowel movements, ideally about 30 minutes after eating. Holland and Frames (1996) also recommend changing the angle between the rectum and anus by using a footstool or altering the height of the toilet seat.

*Weakness of upper extremities*; *fatigue*; and *speech problems* (dysarthria) are other disabling symptoms of multiple sclerosis. Women with severe multiple sclerosis may also have difficulty swallowing. Treatment options for these symptoms include medication, exercise, adaptations in everyday living, and counseling.

# SEXUAL FUNCTIONING

Multiple sclerosis can have both neurological and psychological effects on a woman's sexual functioning. More than 70% of women with multiple sclerosis indicate that their sexuality has been affected (Schapiro: 1994). The neurological effects include reduced sensation in the vagina, decreased vaginal lubrication, and diminished orgasmic response. Spasticity may make some positions difficult or uncomfortable. Bowel or bladder incontinence may cause embarrassment and shame. Partners should know the effects of multiple sclerosis on sexual functioning so that they do not interpret responses as a loss of affection.

Some women are relieved when diagnosed with multiple sclerosis, because the diagnosis may help to explain sexual problems. However, the diagnosis may also affect their self-image severely. In some cases, both women with multiple sclerosis and their partners may reduce physical contact to avoid a possible failure in intimacy and the need to experiment with new positions. Health care professionals should ask routinely about sexual functioning to provide the opportunity for women and their partners to discuss any problems. Shuman and Schwartz (1988) report that some individuals feel as though they are sexual beginners when alternate methods of sexual functioning are suggested.

Women should discuss their medications with physicians to determine how they may affect sexual functioning. Some medications cause drowsiness and lethargy unconducive to sexual performance. Changes in the medications themselves or the schedule for taking the medications may solve sexual functioning problems. Mattson et al. (1995) report that patients who took corticosteroids prescribed for the alleviation of multiple sclerosis symptoms such as numbness, spasticity, fatigue, depression, and pain, experienced improvement in sexual function. Some women with multiple sclerosis find that they have more sexual energy during the morning. Others find that taking medication shortly before intercourse reduces the chance of muscle spasms and relieves their anxiety about having spasms. Experimenting with different positions for intercourse may also reduce spasticity. Women who take drugs to combat fatigue should schedule them before sexual intercourse. Bladder and bowel incontinence may be avoided by reducing fluids and emptying the bladder and bowels prior to intercourse. An in-dwelling bladder catheter may be taped out of the way. Women with vaginal dryness are advised to use commercial, water soluble lubricants.

As is the case with many couples in which a partner develops a disability, communication patterns before onset of disability may be used to predict communication patterns after the onset of disability. Those who have a stable relationship and good communication patterns are often more willing to discuss their needs and experiment to solve sexual problems emanating from the disability. More than two-thirds of individuals with multiple sclerosis who discussed their sexual problems with their spouses and four of six who entered into formal counseling found these discussions helpful (Mattson et al.: 1995). Single women with multiple sclerosis face issues such as finding a partner and disclosing their illness prior to becoming intimate. Many avoid making a commitment for fear that the relationship will be affected by their condition.

Women with multiple sclerosis who are having difficulties with their sexual relationships should consider sexual therapy. If they find communicating with their partners difficult, a third party may help them understand how to continue a fulfilling sexual relationship. Talking with others, even on as sensitive a subject as sexual functioning, can help open the lines of communication, reduce feelings of isolation, and provide information about alternatives that have been helpful to others.

# FAMILY PLANNING, PREGNANCY, AND CHILDREARING

Fertility is unaffected by multiple sclerosis, and women with multiple sclerosis may use the same birth control measures used by healthy women. Oral contraceptives do not affect the incidence of disease flares (Lechtenberg: 1995). The use of barrier methods of contraception such as diaphragms may be difficult if the woman experiences problems with spasticity.

In the past, some physicians routinely recommended that women with multiple sclerosis terminate pregnancies or undergo surgical sterilization (Segal: 1991). However, the long term course of multiple sclerosis seems to be unaffected by pregnancy. Fetal health is also unaffected. There is an increased risk of postpartum flares during the months after delivery. A flare of symptoms may require help from family, friends, or paid assistants in order to perform child care.

Couples should consider the woman's functional level prior to pregnancy. Since it is impossible to predict the course of the disease at the time of diagnosis, it may be prudent to delay childbearing for several years to see if significant disability develops. There is no reason that a woman with severe disease should not have children, but she should consider the physical demands that mothering will make on her. It is also important to assess the potential for stress on the partner due to the extra duties necessitated by the woman's fatigue during pregnancy. If the mother cannot continue to work during pregnancy, will the partner's income be sufficient? How will the couple handle the physical duties of child care, such as lifting, bathing, and carrying the infant? If the mother plans to return to work in about two months, she faces the increased risk of postpartum flares. She must determine if options such as part-time work, working at home, or a leave of absence are available.

In addition to standard obstetrical care, the obstetrician should consult with the woman's neurologist. The anesthesiologist should also be aware of the mother's multiple sclerosis and discuss anesthesia options with the woman. Some women may experience muscle spasms during labor, occasionally requiring a cesarean delivery. The erratic schedule of breastfeeding and infant care, coupled with an increased risk of postpartum flares, may significantly increase fatigue in women with multiple sclerosis. Child care assistance will reduce the stress on mother, father, and infant.

Women with visual impairment due to multiple sclerosis will find many books on child care topics available on "Talking Books," available from the National Library Service for the Blind and Physically Handicapped (see "PUBLICATIONS AND TAPES" section below).

Miller (1992) recommends that health care professionals be prepared to employ the following strategies for easing relations in the families of women with multiple sclerosis. Information about the disease should be provided to children who may be uneasy asking direct questions. Referrals for family therapy should be made if problems are observed. Many families find that support group participation strengthens family dynamics. The National Multiple Sclerosis Society publishes several booklets that provide support to family members (see "PUBLICATIONS AND TAPES" section below) and can make referrals to support programs.

## PSYCHOLOGICAL ASPECTS OF MULTIPLE SCLEROSIS

From the onset of symptoms of multiple sclerosis, the course of the disease is fraught with uncertainty and unpredictability. The unpredictability of multiple sclerosis and the fact that individuals with the disease have a nearly normal life expectancy (Scheinberg: 1983) require continual adjustment and readjustment. The unpredictability of exacerbations is very frustrating.

Women must plan their daily living and work schedules to accommodate the effects of the condition. For example, exacerbations often cause fatigue, which interferes with normal activities, including employment. Women must find a balance between activity and rest periods. Not surprisingly, women who are experiencing exacerbations express higher levels of emotional disturbances than those who are in remission (Warren et al.: 1991).

Fears about the future are to be expected, given the unpredictable course of the disease and the serious consequences that may ensue. Family members may often find that they are taking on additional responsibilities for running the household and making important decisions, resulting in a role reversal between the woman and her partner. Women in strong relationships often find the relationship a source of strength and support to help them cope with the condition (Rodgers and Calder: 1990). At the same time, multiple sclerosis may add a strain to the relationship, including sexual problems. Counseling for both the woman with multiple sclerosis and other family members is often beneficial. Often ignored by health care professionals, the caregiving partner should receive advice on respite care and supportive counseling (White et al.: 1993). However, professional counselors themselves sometimes have fears about the disease that must be addressed in order to provide counseling that meets their clients' psychological needs (Segal: 1991).

In addition to the many physical adaptations required by multiple sclerosis, about half of all individuals with multiple sclerosis experience cognitive problems (Mahler: 1992; Rao et al.: 1991) and must take measures to overcome these difficulties. Among these difficulties are memory problems, concept formation, and depression. These intellectual losses, added to the physical symptoms of multiple sclerosis, may be devastating to the woman's self-esteem and affect social functioning as well as physical activities. Rao and colleagues (1991) found that individuals with multiple sclerosis who had cognitive problems were less likely to be employed and to engage in social activities than individuals without cognitive impairments, even though the severity of physical problems and the duration of the disease were similar for both groups. A study by Sullivan and colleagues (1990) found that most individuals who experienced memory loss and forgetfulness used simple aids such as notepads or daily agendas to keep abreast of their daily needs and schedules. If there are visual problems, large print or a tape recorder may be used to record information.

Symptoms such as stumbling, dropping items, incontinence, and slurred speech may lead to self-consciousness, anxiety, and depression. The woman's personal coping mechanisms and the support provided by family, friends, and the community are crucial to the active problem solving required in living with multiple sclerosis (Shuman and Schwartz: 1988). Women who exhibit these symptoms may also benefit from individual or group counseling.

## PROFESSIONAL SERVICE PROVIDERS

The unique symptoms of each woman with multiple sclerosis require individualized treatment plans. The physical and emotional needs of each woman are best served through a team approach involving medical, allied health, and rehabilitation professionals.

*Neurologists*, who specialize in diseases and conditions of the brain and central nervous system, conduct neurological examinations and interpret the results of tests such as MRIs to diagnose multiple sclerosis and to rule out other possible conditions. *Physiatrists*, or rehabilitation physicians, design an individual treatment plan for patients with multiple sclerosis.

*Physical therapists* teach women with multiple sclerosis how to perform a range of exercises which help build endurance and strength. Physical therapists also prescribe therapeutic exercises to diminish or eliminate weakness, spasticity, and lack of coordination. Physical therapists provide training in the use of assistive devices such as canes, crutches, and orthoses. *Occupational therapists* assess functioning in activities of everyday living and teach simplified techniques of accomplishing them. They may recommend adaptations to the home and work environments. Occupational therapists also suggest adaptive recreation equipment and programs. They can suggest techniques for infant care that will help reduce the added fatigue caused by the physical duties of mothering.

*Orthotists* make and fit assistive devices (orthoses) for improving gait in women with multiple sclerosis. Orthotists, physical therapists, or occupational therapists provide instruction in the use of these devices, such as ankle or foot braces.

*Social workers* provide information about financial and medical benefits, housing, and community resources. They conduct individual, family, or group counseling and may refer individuals to self-help or peer counseling groups.

*Rehabilitation counselors* help individuals with multiple sclerosis develop a plan that will enable them to continue functioning and working. Some individuals will need assistance in returning to their previous position or retraining to obtain a different type of position.

*Psychologists* provide therapy for women and families living with multiple sclerosis. Depression and burnout, for example, may be reduced through marital therapy, helping the couple to balance each other's needs.

*Low vision specialists* may be ophthalmologists, optometrists, opticians, or other professionals trained to help individuals with vision loss use their remaining vision to the greatest extent possible with the assistance of optical and nonoptical aids.

## WHERE TO FIND SERVICES

Neurologists work in private practices, acute care hospitals, and specialty clinics. Neurologists and other members of the multidisciplinary team may also work in transitional or independent living programs and in rehabilitation hospitals. In addition to medical services, MS Comprehensive Care Centers provide services such as physical and occupational therapy, counseling, and patient and family education. A list of these centers is available from the National Multiple Sclerosis Society (see "ORGANIZATIONS" section below). Women who have mobility problems and difficulty traveling to professional service providers' offices often may obtain services in their homes from physical and occupational therapists. Low vision services are often available in ophthalmologists' or optometrists' offices, in private or public agencies that serve individuals who are visually impaired or blind, or in independent practices.

## ASSISTIVE DEVICES AND ENVIRONMENTAL ADAPTATIONS

Women with multiple sclerosis use a combination of environmental adaptations and assistive devices to make everyday routines easier. When making plans for living arrangements or for travel, they must consider a variety of alternatives in the event that their functional abilities deteriorate. For instance, in purchasing a home, it is wise to determine if there is room for a wheelchair ramp.

Some women with gait problems use a cane, crutches, walker, wheelchair, scooter, or a combination of these mobility aids. A woman who usually uses a cane or crutches may prefer to use a wheelchair or scooter when traveling long distances. Special controls installed on cars with automatic transmissions enable many women with multiple sclerosis to continue driving. The gas and brake pedals are operated by hand. These attachments do not interfere with the foot pedals used by other family members. Rehabilitation hospitals and centers offer driver evaluation services such as clinical testing and observation to determine an individual's need for adaptive equipment or training. Major automobile manufacturers offer reimbursement for adaptive equipment installed on new vehicles. (See Chapter 2, "ORGANIZATIONS," page 85 for a listing of programs that offer adaptive equipment for automobiles.)

Heat and humidity affect many women with multiple sclerosis. Air conditioning helps to reduce fatigue and weakness. Physicians, rehabilitation counselors, or tax advisers may provide advice on whether the purchase of an air conditioner is a tax-deductible expense.

A referral to a low vision rehabilitation center offers women with vision problems the opportunity to improve visual function with low vision aids. An eye patch may reduce double vision. Prisms mounted on the eyeglasses lens will expand the visual field of the eye that is not patched. Sunglasses reduce glare and improve contrast for women with optic neuritis. Nonoptical aids such as large print, tape recorders, and high contrast markings are also useful.

Bathtub rails, elevated toilet seats, and grab bars are useful bathroom safety devices. A stall shower is safer and easier to use than a combination tub/shower. A shower chair or tub seat provides additional safety. A hand-held shower attachment is useful when seated.

Some women use assistive devices for dressing, including elastic shoelaces, velcro closures, and buttoning aids. National mail order companies offer clothes that open in front and have reinforced seams, elastic waistbands, and buttons sewn with elastic thread. Formerly these items were limited to leisure and hospital wear, but manufacturers are now designing suits, outerwear, and dressy items for working women who have disabilities. Foam hair rollers, water pipe foam insulation, or layers of tape are used to build up the handles of items as varied as toothbrushes, pens, pencils, eating utensils, paint brushes, and crochet hooks. Remote controls turn on and off lights and televisions and open and close garage doors. Voice dialer telephones permit the storage of frequently called telephone numbers and automatic dialing. A speaker phone allows women with poor motor control or tremors to carry on a telephone conversation comfortably. (See Chapter 2, "VENDORS OF ASSISTIVE DEVICES," page 81 for sources of these devices.)

Computer technology can enable women with multiple sclerosis to continue working and living independently. Screen readers or large print software, keyguards used to prevent unwanted keystrokes, and specially designed keyboards and word prediction software for individuals with limited dexterity are useful adaptations.

References

Calvano, Margaret
1991   Facts & Issues New York, NY: National Multiple Sclerosis Society
1989   Facts & Issues  New York, NY: National Multiple Sclerosis Society
Goodkin, Donald E.
1994   "Interferon Beta-Ib" The Lancet 344:8929:1057
Holland, Nancy and Robin Frames
1996   Understanding Bowel Problems in MS New York, NY: National Multiple Sclerosis Society
Lechtenberg, Richard
1995   Multiple Sclerosis Fact Book  Philadelphia, PA: F. A. Davis Company
Mahler, M. E.
1992   "Behavioral Manifestations Associated with Multiple Sclerosis" Psychiatric Clinics of North America 15(June)2:425-438
Mattson, David et al.
1995   "Multiple Sclerosis: Sexual Dysfunction and Its Response to Medications" Archives of Neurology 52:(September):862-868
Miller, Deborah
1992   "Some Effects of MS On Parenting and Children" pp. 9-24 in Rosalind C. Kalb and Labe C. Scheinberg (eds.) Multiple Sclerosis and the Family New York, NY: Demos Publications

Minden, Sarah L. and Debra Frankel

1989    PLAINTALK: A Booklet About Multiple Sclerosis For Family Members  New York, NY: National Multiple Sclerosis Society

National Center for Health Statistics, Collins, John G.

1988    "Prevalence of Selected Chronic Conditions, United States, 1983-85" Advance Data From Vital and Health Statistics  No. 155 DHHS Pub. No (PHS) 88-1250.  Public Health Service Hyattsville, MD

National Institute of Neurological Disorders and Stroke

1990    Multiple Sclerosis: 1990 Research Program  Bethesda, MD: National Institutes of Health

National Multiple Sclerosis Society

1995    "Expansion of Treatment IND Program for Copolymer 1 (Copaxone)" Research & Medical Programs Department News January 6

Rao, S. M. et al.

1991    "Cognitive Dysfunction in Multiple Sclerosis  II. Impact on Employment and Social Functioning" Neurology  41(May)5:692-696

Reingold, Stephen C.

1996    "New Terms for MS Types" Inside MS  Fall

Rodgers, Jennifer and Peter Calder

1990    "Marital Adjustment:  A Valuable Resource for the Emotional Health of Individuals with Multiple Sclerosis" Rehabilitation Counseling Bulletin 34(September)1:24-32

Schapiro, Randall

1994    Symptom Management in Multiple Sclerosis New York, NY: Demos Publications, Inc.

Scheinberg, Labe

1983    "Signs, Symptoms, and Course of MS" pp. 35-43 in Labe C. Scheinberg (ed.) Multiple Sclerosis: A Guide for Patients and Their Families  New York, NY: Raven Press

Scheinberg, Labe and Charles R. Smith

1989    Rehabilitation of Patients with Multiple Sclerosis  New York, NY: National Multiple Sclerosis Society

Segal, Julia

1991    "Counselling People with Multiple Sclerosis and Their Families" pp. 147-160 in Hilton Davis and Lesley Fallowfield (eds.) Counselling and Communication in Health Care  London: John Wiley and Sons

Shuman, Robert and Janice Schwartz

1988    Understanding Multiple Sclerosis Riverside, NJ: MacMillan Publishing Company

Smith, Charles R. and Labe Scheinberg

1985    "Clinical Features of Multiple Sclerosis" Seminars in Neurology 5(June)2:85-93

Sullivan, Michael J., L. Krista Edgley, and Eric Dehoux

1990    "A Survey of Multiple Sclerosis  Part 1: Perceived Cognitive Problems and Compensatory Strategy Use" Canadian Journal of Rehabilitation 4:2:99-105

Warren, S., K. G. Warren, and R. Cockrill

1991    "Emotional Stress and Coping in Multiple Sclerosis Exacerbations" Journal of Psychosomatic Research 35:1:37-47

White, David M., Marci L. Catanzaro, and George H. Kraft

1993    "An Approach to the Psychological Aspects of Multiple Sclerosis: A Coping Guide for Healthcare Providers and Families" Journal of Neurological Rehabilitation 7:2:43-52

# ORGANIZATIONS

Avonex Support Line
(800) 456-2255                          http://www.biogen.com

Provides information on Avonex, a drug that has recently been approved for treating multiple sclerosis, distribution options, insurance reimbursement counseling, and/or training for self-administration. Phone lines open Monday through Friday, 8:30 a.m. to 8:00 p.m., Eastern Standard Time.

Betaseron Foundation
4828 Parkway Plaza Boulevard, Suite 120
Charlotte, NC 28217-1969
(800) 948-5777

Provides Betaseron, a drug that has recently been approved for treating multiple sclerosis, to qualified underinsured patients. Requirements include a confirmed diagnosis of multiple sclerosis, prescription for Betaseron, inadequate medical insurance, and a Social Security number. Patient financial contribution is required (up to $50.00 per month). Uninsured patients will be referred to Berlex, the manufacturer of Betaseron, for assistance [(800) 788-1467].

MS Pathways
Betaseron
PO Box 52171
Phoenix, AZ 85072-2171
(800) 788-1467                          http://www.betaseron.com

This program provides information on Betaseron, a drug that has recently been approved for treating multiple sclerosis, self-administration training, insurance reimbursement, community support groups, and online services. Publishes quarterly newsletter, "MessageS."

Multiple Sclerosis Society of Canada
250 Bloor Street, East, Suite 1000
Toronto, Ontario M4W 3P9 Canada
(416) 922-6065                In Canada, (800) 268-7582          FAX (416) 922-7538
e-mail: info@mssoc.ca

A national membership organization that funds research, promotes public education, encourages social action on behalf of individuals with multiple sclerosis, and produces many public and professional publications in English and French. The "ASK MS Information System" database of articles on a wide variety of topics, including treatment, research, and social services, is available to people with multiple sclerosis, family members, and health care professionals. Regional divisions and chapters located throughout Canada. National membership, $12.00, Canadian funds; includes newsletter "MS Canada." Membership is free to individuals with multiple sclerosis who live in Canada.

National Association for Continence (NAFC)
PO Box 8310
Spartanburg, SC 29305-8310
(800) 252-3337                          (864) 579-7900                          FAX (864) 579-7902
http://www.nafc.org


An information clearinghouse for consumers, family members, and medical professionals. Will answer individual questions if self-addressed stamped envelope is enclosed with letter. Membership, $15.00, includes a quarterly newsletter, "Quality Care," and a "Resource Guide: Products and Services for Continence" (nonmembers, $15.00). Free publications list.


National Institute of Neurological Disorders and Stroke (NINDS)
Building 31, Room 8A06
31 Center Drive, MSC 2540
Bethesda, MD 20892-2540
(800) 352-9424                          (301) 496-5751                          FAX (301) 402-2186
http://www.ninds.nih.gov


A federal agency which conducts basic and clinical research on the causes and treatment of multiple sclerosis.


National Multiple Sclerosis Society
733 Third Avenue
New York, NY 10017-3288
(212) 986-3240                          FAX (212) 986-7981
(800) 532-7667 Information Resource Center and Library
e-mail: Nat@nmss.org                    http://www.nmss.org


Offers information and referral, counseling services, physician referrals, advocacy, discount prescription and health care products program, and assistance in obtaining adaptive equipment. Provides professional and public education and supports research. Regional affiliates throughout the U.S. Information Resource Center and Library answers telephone inquiries Monday through Thursday, 11:00 a.m. to 5:00 p.m., Eastern Standard Time. Membership, $20.00, includes quarterly large print newsletter, "Inside MS." Individuals with multiple sclerosis may receive a courtesy membership if they are unable to pay.


Shared Solutions
Teva Marion Partners
PO Box 195
Langhorne, PA 19047
(800) 867-2444


This program, sponsored by Teva Marion Partners pharmaceutical company, provides information about multiple sclerosis, treatment reimbursement programs, and local resources.

Simon Foundation for Continence
PO Box 815
Wilmette, IL 60091
(800) 237-4666                    (708) 864-3913                    FAX (708) 864-9758

Provides information and assistance to people who are incontinent. Organizes self-help groups. Membership, individuals, $15.00; professionals, $35.00; includes quarterly newsletter, "The Informer."

ADA and People with MS
by Laura Cooper and Nancy Law with Jane Sarnoff
National Multiple Sclerosis Society
733 Third Avenue
New York, NY 10017-3288
(212) 986-3240                         FAX (212) 986-7981
(800) 532-7667 Information Resource Center and Library
e-mail: Nat@nmss.org                   http://www.nmss.org

This booklet explains how the Americans with Disabilities Act applies to individuals with multiple sclerosis.  Large print.  $.50 plus $2.00 shipping and handling.

Adaptive Parenting Equipment: Idea Book I
Through the Looking Glass
2198 Sixth Street, #100
Berkeley, CA 94710-2204
(800) 644-2666                    (510) 848-1112                    FAX (510) 848-4445
e-mail: tlg@lookingglass.org      http://www.lookingglass.org

A book that describes 50 products to help women with disabilities diaper, bathe, dress, feed, and play with their babies.  Individuals, $10.00; organizations, $25.00.

Aqua Exercise for Multiple Sclerosis
National Multiple Sclerosis Society
733 Third Avenue
New York, NY 10017-3288
(212) 986-3240                         FAX (212) 986-7981
(800) 532-7667 Information Resource Center and Library
e-mail: Nat@nmss.org                   http://www.nmss.org

This videotape presents exercises for building strength and endurance as well as reducing spasticity.  Includes print reference card.  15 minutes.  $17.00.

dirty details, the days and nights of a well spouse
by Marion Deutsche Cohen
Temple University Press
1601 North Broad Street
Philadelphia, PA 19122-6099
(800) 447-1656                    FAX (215) 204-4719
e-mail: tempress@astro.ocis.temple.edu

A frank, personal account, written by a woman whose husband has multiple sclerosis, this book describes her caregiving experiences. Hardcover, $49.95; softcover, $16.95; plus $4.00 shipping and handling.

Employment Issues and Multiple Sclerosis
by Phillip D. Rumrill
Demos Vermande
386 Park Avenue South, Suite 201
New York, NY 10016
(800) 532-8663                    (212) 683-0072                    FAX (212) 683-0118

This book discuss how employment may be affected by multiple sclerosis. Includes information about vocational rehabilitation, job placement and retention, the Americans with Disabilities Act, and other legal issues. $29.95 plus $4.00 shipping and handling.

Enabling Romance: A Guide to Love, Sex, and Relationships for the Disabled
by Ken Kroll and Erica Levy Klein
Woodbine House
6510 Bells Mill Road
Bethesda, MD 20817
(800) 843-7323                    (301) 897-3570                    FAX (301) 897-5838
e-mail: woodbine85@aol.com

Written by a man who has a disability and his wife who does not, this book provides examples of how people with a variety of disabilities have established fulfilling relationships. $15.95 plus $4.00 shipping and handling.

Facts and Issues
National Multiple Sclerosis Society
733 Third Avenue
New York, NY 10017-3288
(212) 986-3240                    FAX (212) 986-7981
(800) 532-7667 Information Resource Center and Library
e-mail: Nat@nmss.org                    http://www.nmss.org

A series of short reports on subjects such as pain, fatigue, and other issues of concern to individuals with multiple sclerosis. Large print. Single copies, $.20 each plus $2.00 shipping and handling.

Fall Down Seven Times Get Up Eight $24.95
Mastering Multiple Sclerosis: A Handbook of Management $24.95
Vignettes: Stories of Life with MS $24.95
by John K. Wolf
Academy Press
PO Box 757
Rutland, VT 05702
(800) 356-3002                    FAX (802) 773-6892

"Fall Down Seven Times Get Up Eight" discusses the effects of multiple sclerosis on everyday living, stress, memory loss, and fatigue. "Mastering Multiple Sclerosis" describes the medical aspects of multiple sclerosis and how to manage its symptoms. "Vignettes" is a collection of essays, poems, and stories by and about individuals with multiple sclerosis.

Frank Talk
by JoAnn LeMaistre
Alpine Guild
PO Box 4846
Dillon, CO 80435
(800) 869-9559                    FAX (970) 262-9378

In this videotape, individuals with multiple sclerosis share their concerns about living with chronic illness and discuss coping strategies.  30 minutes.  $39.95

Intermittent Self-Catheterization
Media Services
Sacred Heart Medical Center
PO Box 2555
Spokane, WA 99220-2555
(509) 458-5236                    FAX (509) 626-4475

This videotape demonstrates the use of sterile techniques for intermittent catheterization and shows the necessary supplies and procedures.  8 minutes.  Purchase, $135.00; rental for one week, $45.00 (may be applied toward purchase); plus $5.00 shipping and handling.

Living Well with MS: A Guide for Patient, Caregiver, and Family
by David L. Carroll and Jon Dudley Dorman
Harper Collins Publishers
PO Box 588
Dunmore, PA 18512
(800) 331-3761                    http://www.harpercollins.com/

In addition to information on multiple sclerosis and its diagnosis, prognosis, and treatment, this book discusses emotional and sexual functioning.  $12.00 plus $2.75 shipping and handling.

Living with Low Vision: A Resource Guide for People with Sight Loss
Resources for Rehabilitation
33 Bedford Street, Suite 19A
Lexington, MA 02173
(617) 862-6455                    FAX (617) 861-7517

This resource guide directs people who have experienced vision loss to services, products, and publications that enable them to keep reading, working, and enjoying life.  Large print.  $43.95 plus $5.00 shipping and handling.  (See order form on last page of this book.)

Living with Multiple Sclerosis: A New Handbook for Families
by Robert Shuman and Janice Schwartz
MacMillan Publishing Company
201 West 103rd Street
Indianapolis, IN 46290
(800) 428-5331

In this book, two psychologists discuss the role of the family with a member who has multiple sclerosis. Includes chapters on adolescents with multiple sclerosis, employment, and research. Uses real life experiences to suggest coping strategies and adaptations. $10.00 plus $3.00 shipping and handling.

Living with Multiple Sclerosis: A Wellness Approach
by George H. Kraft and Marci Catanzaro
Demos Vermande
386 Park Avenue South, Suite 201
New York, NY 10016
(800) 532-8663                    (212) 683-0072                    FAX (212) 683-0118

This book suggest strategies for everyday living with multiple sclerosis. Includes information on diet, nutrition, and exercise. $13.95 plus $4.00 shipping and handling.

Managing Incontinence
Cheryle B. Gartley, (ed.)
Simon Foundation for Continence
PO Box 815
Wilmette, IL 60091
(800) 237-4666                    (708) 864-3913                    FAX (708) 864-9758

This book provides medical advice, information on products, interviews with individuals who are incontinent, and advice on sexuality. $11.95

Mother-to-Be: A Guide to Pregnancy and Birth For Women with Disabilities
by Judith Rogers and Molleen Matsumura
Demos Vermande
386 Park Avenue South, Suite 201
New York, NY 10016
(800) 532-8663                    (212) 683-0072                    FAX (212) 683-0118

This book describes the pregnancy and childbirth experiences of 36 women with a wide variety of disabilities including multiple sclerosis. Suggests practical solutions for the special concerns of women with disabilities during pregnancy and those of their partners, families, and health care providers. Includes a list of resources, glossary, and bibliography. $24.95 plus $4.00 shipping and handling.

Moving with Multiple Sclerosis: An Exercise Manual for People with Multiple Sclerosis
by Iris Kimberg
National Multiple Sclerosis Society
733 Third Avenue
New York, NY 10017-3288
(212) 986-3240                    FAX (212) 986-7981
(800) 532-7667 Information Resource Center and Library
e-mail: Nat@nmss.org                    http://www.nmss.org

This booklet describes four types of exercises designed to relieve some multiple sclerosis symptoms. Includes passive range of motion and stretching, active and active restrictive, coordination and balance, and exercises to reduce spasticity. Numerous illustrations guide a woman and a helper through each exercise sequence. Large print. $1.50 plus $2.00 shipping and handling.

**Multiple Sclerosis: A Guide for Patients and Their Families**
by Labe C. Scheinberg and Nancy J. Holland
Raven Press
PO Box 1600
Hagerstown, MD 21741
(800) 777-2295       (301) 714-2300       FAX (301) 824-7390
http://www.ravenpress.com

Written by physicians, nurses, an occupational therapist, a social worker, a rehabilitation counselor, and others, this book provides basic information on the causes and course of multiple sclerosis, vocational choices, disability benefits, sexuality, and community resources. Hardcover, $27.50; softcover, $17.00; plus $4.50 shipping and handling.

**Multiple Sclerosis: A Guide for the Newly Diagnosed**
by Nancy Holland, T. Jock Murray, and Stephen Reingold
Demos Vermande
386 Park Avenue South, Suite 201
New York, NY 10016
(800) 532-8663       (212) 683-0072       FAX (212) 683-0118

This book provides information about multiple sclerosis and medical treatments as well as its effect on the individual and the family. $21.95 plus $4.00 shipping and handling.

**Multiple Sclerosis and the Family**
by Rosalind C. Kalb and Labe C. Scheinberg (eds.)
Demos Vermande
386 Park Avenue South, Suite 201
New York, NY 10016
(800) 532-8663       (212) 683-0072       FAX (212) 683-0118

Written for individuals with multiple sclerosis, their families, and health professionals, this book describes the impact of multiple sclerosis on the family and recommends resources and strategies for living with the disease. Includes chapters on family planning, pregnancy, parenting, and sexuality. $24.95 plus $4.00 shipping and handling.

**Multiple Sclerosis: A Rehabilitation Approach to Management**
by Randall T. Schapiro
Demos Vermande
386 Park Avenue South, Suite 201
New York, NY 10016
(800) 532-8663       (212) 683-0072       FAX (212) 683-0118

This book discusses the rehabilitation techniques and roles of health professionals who work with individuals who have multiple sclerosis. Includes psychological, social, and family issues. $21.95 plus $4.00 shipping and handling.

Multiple Sclerosis Fact Book
by Richard Lechtenberg
F.A. Davis Company
1915 Arch Street
Philadelphia, PA 19103
(800) 323-3555                  In AK and HI, (215) 440-3001      FAX (215) 440-3016
e-mail: orders@fadavis.com      http://www.fadavis.com

Written for the lay person, this book describes up-to-date diagnostic tests and therapies and provides practical ideas for coping with multiple sclerosis. $19.95

Multiple Sclerosis Quarterly Report
Demos Vermande
386 Park Avenue South, Suite 201
New York, NY 10016
(800) 532-8663                  (212) 683-0072                  FAX (212) 683-0118

This newsletter reports advances in the diagnosis and treatment of multiple sclerosis. $16.00.

Multiple Sclerosis: The Questions You Have, The Answers You Need
by Rosalind Kalb (ed.)
Demos Vermande
386 Park Avenue South, Suite 201
New York, NY 10016
(800) 532-8663                  (212) 683-0072                  FAX (212) 683-0118

Written by professionals who care for individuals with multiple sclerosis, this book provides information about living with the condition and answers questions most commonly asked. Topics include neurology, treatment, employment, legal issues, physical and occupational therapy, psychosocial issues, sexuality, and reproductive health. $39.95 plus $4.00 shipping and handling.

The Other Victim - Caregivers Share Their Coping Strategies
by Alan Drattell
Seven Locks Press
PO Box 25689
Santa Ana, CA 92799
(800) 354-5348

This book is a collection of personal accounts of nine caregivers of individuals with multiple sclerosis. Also includes a resource list of organizations and suggestions for coping. $17.95 plus $4.00 shipping and handling.

PLAINTALK: A Booklet About Multiple Sclerosis For Family Members
by Sarah L. Minden and Debra Frankel
National Multiple Sclerosis Society
733 Third Avenue
New York, NY 10017-3288
(212) 986-3240                    FAX (212) 986-7981
(800) 532-7667 Information Resource Center and Library
e-mail: Nat@nmss.org              http://www.nmss.org

This booklet simulates a support group meeting for families of individuals with multiple sclerosis. Discusses diagnosis, everyday living, talking with children, and the well parent. Large print. $.55 plus $2.00 shipping and handling.

Providing Services for People with Vision Loss: A Multidisciplinary Perspective
by Susan L. Greenblatt (ed.)
Resources for Rehabilitation
33 Bedford Street, Suite 19A
Lexington, MA 02173
(617) 862-6455                    FAX (617) 861-7517

This anthology discusses how health and rehabilitation professionals can work together to provide coordinated care for individuals who have experienced vision loss. Also available on audiocassette. $19.95 plus $5.00 shipping and handling. (See order form on last page of this book.)

Real Living with Multiple Sclerosis
Springhouse Corporation
1111 Bethlehem Pike
Springhouse, PA 19477
(800) 783-4903

This monthly publication provides information about research and medical treatment as well as support through personal experiences and tips for everyday living with multiple sclerosis. $49.00

Reproductive Issues for Persons with Physical Disabilities
by Florence P. Haseltine, Sandra S. Cole, and David B. Gray (eds.)
Brookes Publishing Company
PO Box 10624
Baltimore, MD 21285-9945
(800) 638-3775                    e-mail: custserv@p.brookes.com

This book provides an overview of sexuality, disability, and reproductive issues across the lifespan for individuals with disabilities including multiple sclerosis. Includes academic articles as well as personal narratives written by individuals with disabilities. $34.00

Sexual Dysfunction
by Robin Frames
National Multiple Sclerosis Society
733 Third Avenue
New York, NY 10017-3288
(212) 986-3240                    FAX (212) 986-7981
(800) 532-7667 Information Resource Center and Library
e-mail: Nat@nmss.org              http://www.nmss.org

This booklet describes how multiple sclerosis may affect women's and men's sexual function. Discusses symptoms and treatment options and suggests coping techniques. Large print. $.45 plus $2.00 shipping and handling.

Someone You Know Has MS: A Book for Families  $.55
by Cyrisse Jaffee, Debra Frankel, Barbara LaRoche and Patricia Dick
When a Parent Has MS: A Teenager's Guide  $.50
by Pamela Cavallo with Martha Jablow
National Multiple Sclerosis Society
733 Third Avenue
New York, NY 10017-3288
(212) 986-3240                    FAX (212) 986-7981
(800) 532-7667 Information Resource Center and Library
e-mail: Nat@nmss.org              http://www.nmss.org

These two booklets, one written for children age 6-12 and the other for teenagers, help youngsters understand their parent's condition and discuss the youngsters' concerns and fears. Large print. Add $2.00 shipping and handling.

Symptom Management in Multiple Sclerosis
by Randall T. Schapiro
Demos Vermande
386 Park Avenue South, Suite 201
New York, NY 10016
(800) 532-8663              (212) 683-0072              FAX (212) 683-0118

A multidisciplinary guide for health care professionals and individuals with multiple sclerosis which suggests management strategies for treating multiple sclerosis and minimizing and controlling its symptoms. $19.95 plus $4.00 shipping and handling.

Taking Care: A Guide for Well Partners
by Nancy J. Holland with Jane Sarnoff
National Multiple Sclerosis Society
733 Third Avenue
New York, NY 10017-3288
(212) 986-3240                    FAX (212) 986-7981
(800) 532-7667 Information Resource Center and Library
e-mail: Nat@nmss.org              http://www.nmss.org

This booklet discusses how to balance the needs of both partners and how to ask for and receive help. Large print. $.40 plus $2.00 shipping and handling.

Talking Books for People with Physical Disabilities
National Library Service for the Blind and Physically Handicapped (NLS)
1291 Taylor Street, NW
Washington, DC 20542
(800) 424-8567 or (800) 424-8572 (Reference Section)
(800) 424-9100 (to receive application)
(202) 707-5100                    FAX (202) 707-0712
telnet marvel.loc.gov (log in as marvel, select Library of Congress Online Systems, select connect to LOCIS, then select "Braille and Audio" for a catalogue of braille and tape publications)

This brochure describes a free program which provides books and magazines recorded on discs and audiocassettes for individuals with multiple sclerosis and other disabling conditions. Application forms are available from the NLS, public libraries, or local affiliates of the National Multiple Sclerosis Society. A health professional must certify that the individual is unable to hold a book or turn pages; has blurred or double vision; extreme weakness or excessive fatigue; or other physical limitations which prevent the individual from reading standard print.

Therapeutic Claims in Multiple Sclerosis: A Guide to Treatments
by William A. Sibley
Demos Vermande
386 Park Avenue South, Suite 201
New York, NY 10016
(800) 532-8663                    (212) 683-0072                    FAX (212) 683-0118

In addition to basic information about the symptoms and diagnosis of multiple sclerosis, this book describes the most frequently used therapies and their effectiveness. An opinion statement, made by the International Federation of Multiple Sclerosis Societies, accompanies each listing. $24.95 plus $4.00 shipping and handling.

Understanding Bladder Problems in Multiple Sclerosis
by Nancy J. Holland and Michele G. Madonna
National Multiple Sclerosis Society
733 Third Avenue
New York, NY 10017-3288
(212) 986-3240                    FAX (212) 986-7981
(800) 532-7667 Information Resource Center and Library
e-mail: Nat@nmss.org                    http://www.nmss.org

This booklet describes how multiple sclerosis affects the urinary system; how to control symptoms; and how to manage bladder dysfunction. Large print. $.45 plus $2.00 shipping and handling.

<u>Understanding Bowel Problems in MS</u>
by Nancy J. Holland and Robin Frames
National Multiple Sclerosis Society
733 Third Avenue
New York, NY 10017-3288
(212) 986-3240                          FAX (212) 986-7981
(800) 532-7667 Information Resource Center and Library
e-mail: Nat@nmss.org                    http://www.nmss.org

This booklet describes common bowel problems and suggests coping strategies. Large print. $.45 plus $2.00 shipping and handling.

<u>You Are Not Your Illness</u>
by Linda Noble Topf
Simon and Schuster
200 Old Tappan Road
Old Tappan, NJ 07675
(800) 223-2348                          e-mail: ss cust serv@prenhall.com
http://www.simonsays.com

In this book, the author, who has multiple sclerosis, shares her personal perspectives on living with chronic illness. She describes a step-by-step process for dealing with loss and maintaining feelings of self-worth. $12.00 plus $3.00 shipping and handling.

# Chapter 9

# *OSTEOPOROSIS*

Osteoporosis, a condition in which there is too little bone mass, occurs in one out of every four women over 60 (Palmieri: 1988). Osteoporosis is a major cause of fractures of the spine, hip, and wrist. There are approximately 247,000 hip fractures annually in Americans over 45; one in two women over the age of 65 will experience fractures due to osteoporosis (Lyon and Sutton: 1993). The most common fracture in women age 50 to 74 is a fracture of the forearm (Peck et al.: 1988).

Half of the individuals who experience a hip fracture caused by osteoporosis require some help with daily living, and 15 to 25% enter long term care institutions. The pain and disability associated with osteoporosis have economic consequences that are reflected in medical, nursing home, and social costs. In the United States, these costs are 10 billion dollars and rising (National Osteoporosis Foundation: 1996a).

Although the causes of osteoporosis are not clear, it has been suggested that decreased levels of estrogen and calcium are responsible for weakened bones. Bone strength is also affected by exercise; women who exercise regularly lose less bone mass than those who remain sedentary.

The most susceptible individuals are fair skinned, white women who are thin, have small frames, have a family history of osteoporosis, or have had their ovaries removed at an early age (National Institute on Aging: 1983). A woman who has had her ovaries removed before menopause has severely reduced levels of estrogen; if she does not take estrogen, she is at greater risk for osteoporosis. Other factors associated with the development of osteoporosis are alcohol consumption and cigarette smoking; the use of anti-inflammatory drugs to treat arthritis and lupus, antiepileptic drugs, and blood thinners also increase the risk for osteoporosis. Women who have diabetes lose calcium through excessive urination; kidney dialysis contributes to calcium loss as well. A recent study reported that women over age 55 who were being treated with oral or inhaled corticosteroids had lower bone densities than men who received the same treatment (Marystone et al.: 1995).

Loss of height, which occurs when weakened bones in the spine compress, fracture, and collapse, is an early sign of osteoporosis, but the condition is most often confirmed only through the use of x-rays following a fracture. Conventional x-rays do not adequately measure loss of bone mass, but other procedures do. Single or dual-photon absorptiometry measures bone mineral content, exposing the individual to lower radiation levels than conventional x-rays. The quantitative computed tomography scan (QCT) measures bone tissue. Although bone density tests may be used to detect osteoporosis, predict future fractures, and determine bone loss rates or efficacy of treatment (when conducted at regular intervals), they are expensive and not available to the general population (Earnshaw and Hosking: 1996). (Bone density tests may not be covered by health insurance.)

Compression fractures of the spine may lead to the development of the "dowager's hump," caused by loss of height and rounded shoulders. This condition affects the woman's posture and may make her more susceptible to falls. It may also make the individual more prone to breathing problems, because the chest cavity is compressed. In women with osteoporosis, fractures can even be caused by a sneeze, cough, or hug.

To prevent osteoporosis, experts recommend that women exercise regularly, stop smoking, use caffeine and alcohol moderately, increase the amount of calcium in their daily diet, and consider estrogen replacement after menopause.

Clinical trials supported by the National Institute on Aging are testing new approaches to maintain or increase bone strength in individuals over age 65. The causes of progressive bone loss in later life are also being studied.

The Women's Health Initiative, a major research study being conducted by the National Institutes of Health, is recruiting women, age 50 to 79, to participate in clinical trials evaluating the effects of estrogen replacement therapy and calcium and vitamin D supplements on prevention of fractures caused by osteoporosis (see "ORGANIZATIONS" section below).

## TYPES OF OSTEOPOROSIS

Bone tissue is formed, broken down, resorbed, and replaced throughout life in a process called bone remodeling. Cells called osteoclasts dissolve bone tissue, releasing calcium to be used in other parts of the body. The tissue is replaced by osteoblasts, cells that draw calcium and phosphorus from the bloodstream and deposit them on the bones as collagen. In several weeks the collagen hardens to form new bone. According to Lyon and Sutton (1993), the bone remodeling process replaces nearly one-third of an individual's bone tissue in a year.

Bone tissue grows during childhood, adolescence, and early adulthood, peaking between the age of 15 and 30; after age 35, bone loss overtakes bone replacement. *Postmenopausal osteoporosis*, also referred to as *estrogen-dependent osteoporosis* (Type I), is a phase of rapid bone loss accelerated by menopause; it occurs for a relatively brief period of time and increases the risk of spine and wrist fractures (Persky and Alexander: 1989). Investigators have shown that estrogen has a protective effect on bone which is lost at menopause (National Osteoporosis Foundation: 1989). Both women and men are affected by *age-dependent osteoporosis* (Type II), which occurs in individuals over the age of 65 and makes them susceptible to hip fractures; bone loss occurs more slowly in this type of osteoporosis. *Secondary osteoporosis* is the term used to describe bone loss due to a known cause, such as the side effects of certain medications.

The following factors may help prevent the loss of bone mass and development of osteoporosis:
• *Good nutrition* Calcium plays a major role in the development and maintenance of strong bones. Pregnant women and women who are breastfeeding should increase their intake of calcium, for their own health and their baby's health. The mother's calcium supply will be depleted by the baby's needs, so she should eat foods rich in calcium in order to replenish it. Most adults should consume calcium by eating dairy products and other foods rich in calcium, such as salmon, broccoli, soybeans, and almonds. It is recommended that daily calcium intake in postmenopausal women (age 50-64) who are taking estrogen should be 1000 milligrams; in postmenopausal women not taking estrogen and those age 65 and over, daily calcium intake should be 1,500 milligrams (National Osteoporosis Foundation: 1995). Vitamin D, formed in the body after exposure to sunlight, aids the body in absorbing calcium. Women who do not receive enough sunlight may need a vitamin supplement. A registered dietitian or nutritionist, physician, or pharmacist can advise women which calcium supplements have the best absorption rates, do not interfere with other prescription or over-the-counter medications, and will not lead to excessive calcium intake. Women who wish to lower their fat intake and those who have lactose intolerance may substitute skim and low fat milk and yogurt or products reduced in lactose in order to meet dietary guidelines for calcium intake. Fluoride therapy, which stimulates bone formation and density, is controversial because of undesirable side effects and doubts regarding its effectiveness in preventing hip fractures (Hahn: 1988).
• *Exercise* Walking, jogging, dancing, bicycling, and other forms of weight-bearing exercise are recommended to help decrease bone loss. Simple exercises which promote good posture and muscle strength will also help prevent injuries. Physical therapists caution women with osteoporosis to avoid bending forward during daily activities, which may lead to crush fractures in the spine.

• *Hormone therapy* The number of hip, spine, and wrist fractures is significantly reduced in women on estrogen replacement therapy compared with those women who have never taken the hormone (National Osteoporosis Foundation: 1989). In addition to reducing osteoporosis, hormone replacement therapy has been shown to reduce the risk of cardiovascular disease and aid in maintaining low cholesterol levels. Several studies have indicated a slightly increased risk for endometrial cancer among women who have estrogen therapy. Women who have had certain types of cancer, liver disease, high blood pressure, and other conditions should not take estrogen. Estrogen alone may be taken by women who have had hysterectomies. Estrogen taken with progesterone lowers the risk but may not be as effective in preventing heart disease. Each woman must carefully consider the risks and benefits of estrogen therapy, as well as the duration of treatment. Estrogen or estrogen plus progesterone may be taken as oral medication, or a woman may choose to use a transdermal patch, worn on an inconspicuous part of the body.

• *Calcitonin therapy*, a hormone provided through injection or a nasal spray, has been found to be effective in women with Type I osteoporosis (Avioli: 1992). Although a runny nose is the only side effect reported for the nasal spray form of treatment, allergic reactions, nausea, frequent urination, flushing of the hands and face, and skin reactions are reported side effects of injectable calcitonin (National Osteoporosis Foundation: 1996b).

• *Alendronate therapy* (Fosamax), a nonhormonal prescription medication, has been approved by the Food and Drug Administration for use by women after menopause. In several large studies, individuals taking the drug showed a significant increase in bone mass in the hip and spine (Food and Drug Administration: 1995). Since nausea, heartburn, and irritation of the esophagus are possible side effects, it is recommended that a woman take the medication in the morning on an empty stomach, drinking six to eight ounces of water. She should avoid eating, drinking other beverages, or taking other medications, and she should sit or stand upright for at least 30 minutes to an hour after taking Fosamax, to reduce the risk of these side effects.

## ACCIDENT PREVENTION

It has been estimated that a third of noninstitutionalized individuals age 65 or over fall each year; among elders in long term care facilities, the proportion is higher. In most cases, falls do not cause serious injuries, although more than 215,000 falls each year result in hip fractures (National Institute on Aging: 1991). Hip fractures, in turn, may lead to other health problems and a consequent loss of independence.

Risk factors for falls include the use of sedatives, cognitive impairment, alcohol consumption, and posture and gait problems. In addition to osteoporosis, other conditions found in elders, such as Parkinson's disease, stroke, and visual impairment, are predisposing factors for falls. Environmental hazards are also the source of a large proportion of falls. Many older women have multiple disabilities that are risk factors for falls, and often the exact cause or causes of a given fall are unknown.

Tinetti and her colleagues (1988) found that nearly one-third (32%) of individuals 75 years or older living in the community fell at least once during their one year study. Of those who fell, one-quarter (24%) sustained serious injuries.

Several investigators have suggested that the fear of falling itself results in the self-imposed limitation of activity by many elders (Duthie: 1989; Tinetti et al.: 1988). One study (Walker and Howland: 1991) found that fear of falling resulted in the curtailment of activities by 41% of the respondents.

Ironically, the fear of falling may actually result in additional falls, because inactivity may cause weakness and hinder joint mobility (Sattin: 1992; Walker and Howland: 1991). Research has confirmed that exercise may play a protective role in preventing fractures among elders (National Institute on Aging: 1991; Sorock et al.: 1988). Health care professionals, especially physical therapists, can help develop walking and exercise programs that build muscle strength and enable older women to continue to be active.

Since most falls in the older population occur in the home, environmental adaptations may reduce the occurrence of falls and provide reassurance to women who have fallen in the past and fear falling again. There are many obvious ways of making the home safer and preventing falls; these include using nonskid rugs, providing good lighting and reducing glare, installing grab bars in tubs and next to toilets, using bath chairs in the shower and tub, and eliminating elevated thresholds. Level, nonskid floors, uncluttered halls and aisles, night lights, and handrails along stairs may also help to prevent falls. The use of canes and other mobility aids may assist women who have trouble walking and bolster their confidence as well.

Personal response systems for emergencies may reduce the fear of falling, fostering self-confidence in older women with disabilities and enabling family members or other caregivers to feel comfortable when leaving the home. If a woman falls or experiences symptoms of a medical emergency, she activates the system, usually by pushing a device that is worn around the neck or kept nearby, that alerts a designated response network. Purchase and installation of equipment may be reimbursable by third-party payment, although the individual is usually responsible for monthly service fees.

Public health officials, recognizing that falls among elders pose a serious health problem, have suggested that prevention programs be implemented on a widespread basis. Using the risk factors associated with falling to determine the target population, occupational therapists, architects, and others trained in environmental adaptations could conduct assessments of the home environments of older women as well as places that they frequent, such as senior centers and churches. Checklists of home safety items are available from a number of organizations to facilitate this undertaking (see "PUBLI-CATIONS AND TAPES" section below).

Women who use exercise to maintain strong bones and muscles are less apt to be injured than those who are sedentary. With the following suggestions in mind, older women should perform a safety check of their homes to remove obstacles; they should make other changes to avoid falls and accidents which lead to fractures. Staff members at senior centers and other public areas where elders meet should also be aware of these suggestions:

- Sturdy, low-heeled, soft-soled shoes are safer than high heels with slick soles. Shoes that are too large and slip-on sandals and slippers are also dangerous. Long bathrobes or other full-length garments may result in falls.
- Scatter rugs, loose telephone and electric cords, and clutter should be removed. Nonskid mats should be used in bathtubs and showers, and grab bars should be installed.
- Night-lights should be used in bathrooms and halls, and bright bulbs should be used in stairs and halls.
- Handrails should be installed in stairways, and treads or carpeting used on stairs should be firmly fastened down.
- Caution should be used on wet, icy, uneven, or broken pavement. Curbs, slick floors, tile floors, and oil leaks present hazards to women with osteoporosis.
- Older women should ask their physicians about side effects of medications, such as dizziness, balance problems, or light-headedness. The use of alcohol may also affect balance and reflexes.
- Older women should have their vision and hearing checked regularly. Inadequate refraction for eyeglasses or the build-up of ear wax may cause balance problems.

- Older women should consult with a physical therapist for suggestions to help reduce their risk for fractures. Proper sitting and standing positions, correct pulling and pushing techniques, and reducing stress on the back and joints when sleeping or resting will enable them to live more comfortably with osteoporosis.

## PSYCHOLOGICAL ASPECTS OF OSTEOPOROSIS

Older women with osteoporosis need to consider changes in their lifestyle to reduce the chance of injury. Such changes may include moving to a home or apartment with only one floor in order to avoid falls on stairs; giving up chores which involve heavy lifting; and learning to use assistive devices in everyday activities. Moving to a new environment, giving up normal routines, and finding new friends require psychological adjustments. Fear of falling often results in activity limitation and staying indoors. The social isolation that results may contribute to loneliness and depression. Older women who find themselves depressed by the multiple changes in their lives may wish to seek counseling from a social worker or psychologist or join a self-help group to learn from others in similar situations.

It is not unusual for older women to become depressed when hospitalized or placed in a long term care facility due to a fracture and to be anxious about their future. Daily living with osteoporosis may require that women use medication to cope with pain; receive physical therapy to maintain flexibility; and be very cautious in everyday activities. These factors may affect their motivation to participate in a rehabilitation program.

## PROFESSIONAL SERVICE PROVIDERS

*Gynecologists* often serve as the primary care physicians for women in the age ranges most at risk for osteoporosis. Gynecologists may recommend estrogen replacement therapy for women at menopause, after carefully weighing the benefits and potential risks.

*Orthopedic surgeons* or *plastic surgeons* may perform surgery to repair or replace bones damaged by fractures caused by osteoporosis. Hip or knee replacement surgery may be recommended.

*Physiatrists*, physicians who specialize in rehabilitation medicine, will often first see the individual after a fracture and admission to a rehabilitation program. Physiatrists evaluate the fracture and develop the overall rehabilitation plan. Physiatrists act as case managers, coordinating medical and rehabilitation services, working with the primary care physician, and arranging for physical therapy, if necessary.

*Physical therapists* design individualized programs to improve posture and strengthen muscles. Physical therapists also teach how to move safely to avoid injury.

*Occupational therapists* may perform a home safety assessment, making suggestions for accident prevention, such as removing loose electrical cords and throw rugs, installing grab bars, and increasing lighting in stairways, halls, and bathrooms.

*Registered dietitians* or *nutritionists* recommend dietary measures to ensure that women eat the foods that supply important nutrients for the maintenance of their bones.

*Social workers* help patients with osteoporosis plan for discharge from a hospital or a rehabilitation center to an environment where they can function independently. This may include discharge to the individual's home with arrangements for home health care; to a relative's home; to a long term care facility; or to congregate housing.

Women with osteoporosis will often be hospitalized for corrective surgery when a fracture occurs; when difficult diagnostic procedures are necessary; or for rehabilitation. They may enter a rehabilitation unit within a community hospital or a rehabilitation hospital. Most rehabilitation centers also offer outpatient services.

Women who have had a fracture may require home health services, including home treatment and maintenance care provided by nurses or home health aides; homemaker services such as meal preparation; Meals on Wheels; chore services such as housecleaning; and adult day activity programs. For some, these services may be needed on a short term basis. They are provided by public and private agencies.

Some of the transportation needs of individuals whose everyday functioning has been affected by osteoporosis may be met through the use of special van services or special parking placards for individuals with disabilities.

References

Avioli, Louis V.
1992    "Osteoporosis Syndromes: Patient Selection for Calcitonin Therapy" Geriatrics 47(April)4:58-67

Duthie, Edmund H.
1989    "Falls" Medical Clinics of North America 73(November):6:1321-1336

Earnshaw, S. A. and D. J. Hosking
1996    "Clinical Usefulness of Risk Factors for Osteoporosis" Annals of the Rheumatic Diseases 55:6:338

Food and Drug Administration
1995    "FDA Approves New Drug for Bones Disorders" FDA Talk Paper October 2

Hahn, Bevra H.
1988    "Osteoporosis: Diagnosis and Management" Bulletin on the Rheumatic Diseases 38:1-9 Atlanta, GA: Arthritis Foundation

Lyon, Wanda S. and Cynthia E. Sutton
1993    Osteoporosis: How to Make Your Bones Last a Lifetime Orlando, FL: Tribune Publishing

Marystone, Jane F., Elizabeth L. Barrett-Connor, and Deborah J. Morton
1995    "Inhaled and Oral Corticosteroids: Their Effects on Bone Mineral Density in Older Adults" American Journal of Public Health 85:12:1693

National Institute on Aging
1991    Physical Frailty Department of Health and Human Services, NIH Publication 91-397
1983    "Osteoporosis: The Bone Thinner" Age Page Washington, DC: National Institute on Aging

National Osteoporosis Foundation
1996a Fast Facts on Osteoporosis Washington, DC: National Osteoporosis Foundation
1996b Medications Used to Prevent and Treat Osteoporosis Washington, DC: National Osteoporosis Foundation
1995    Calcium: Important at Every Age Washington, DC: National Osteoporosis Foundation
1989    Boning Up on Osteoporosis Washington, DC: National Osteoporosis Foundation

Palmieri, Genaro M. A.
1988    "Prevention and Treatment of Osteoporosis" Clinical Report on Aging 2:19-20 New York, NY: American Geriatrics Society

Peck, William et al.
1988   "Research Directions in Osteoporosis" <u>The American Journal of Medicine</u> 84(February):275-282

Persky, Neal and Neil Alexander
1989   "Issues of Aging in Preventive Medicine and the Example of Osteoporosis" <u>Primary Care</u> 16(March)1:231-243

Sattin, Richard W.
1992   "Falls among Older Persons:  A Public Health Perspective" <u>Annual Review of Public Health</u> 13:489-508

Sorock, Gary S. et al.
1988   "Physical Activity and Fracture Risk in a Free-Living Elderly Cohort" <u>Journal of Gerontology Medical Sciences</u> 43:5:M134-139

Tinetti, Mary E., Mark Speechley, and Sandra F. Ginter
1988   "Risk Factors for Falls among Elderly Persons Living in the Community" <u>New England Journal of Medicine</u>  349:26:1701-1707

Walker, J. Elizabeth and Jonathan Howland
1991   "Falls and Fear of Falling among Elderly Persons Living in the Community:  Occupational Therapy Interventions" <u>American Journal of Occupational Therapy</u> 45(February):2:119-122

# ORGANIZATIONS

Calcium Information Center
New York Hospital-Cornell Medical Center
515 East 71st Street, F-904
New York, NY 10021
(800) 321-2681

Distributes information about the role of calcium in preventing and treating medical disorders. Responds to individual requests received on toll-free information line.

National Arthritis and Musculoskeletal and Skin Diseases Information Clearinghouse
1 AMS Circle
Bethesda, MD 20892-3675
(301) 495-4484                    (301) 565-296 (TT)                    FAX (301) 587-4352

Distributes information, bibliographies, fact sheets, and catalogues to health care professionals.

National Center for Nutrition and Dietetics
American Dietetic Association
216 West Jackson Boulevard
Chicago, IL 60606-6995
Consumer Nutrition Hot Line (800) 366-1655                    (312) 899-0040
FAX (312) 899-1758                    http://www.eatright.org

Callers may receive a referral to a registered dietitian or listen to recorded nutrition messages in English and Spanish. Customized food and nutrition information from a registered dietitian is available by calling (900) 225-5267; the cost of a call is $1.95 for the first minute, $.95 for each minute thereafter. Free publications.

National Institute of Arthritis and Musculoskeletal and Skin Diseases (NIAMS)
Building 31, Room 4C-32
9000 Rockville Pike
Bethesda, MD 20892
(301) 496-8190                    FAX (301) 480-6069                    http://www.nih.gov/niams

NIAMS supports research on bone disorders, including osteoporosis; provides professional, public, and patient education; and sponsor community activities.

National Osteoporosis Foundation (NOF)
1150 17th Street, NW, Suite 500
Washington, DC 20036
(800) 223-9994                    (202) 223-2226                    FAX (202) 223-2237
http://www.nof.org

Provides public and professional education materials and supports research. Free publications list. Membership, $15.00, includes quarterly newsletter, "The Osteoporosis Report," periodic medical updates, and discounts on educational materials. Materials available in English and Spanish.

Osteoporosis and Related Bone Diseases National Resource Center (ORBD)
1150 17th Street, Suite 500
Washington, DC 20036-4603
(800) 624-2663                    (202) 223-0344                    (202) 466-4315 (TT)
FAX (202) 223-2237               e-mail: orbdnrc@nof.org          http://www.osteo.org

Provides public and professional education materials on metabolic bone diseases including osteoporosis. Makes referrals to physicians and support groups. ORBD will conduct special searches of its databases, BoneData and the Cumulative Index to Metabolic Bone Diseases Literature. Annotated bibliographies on many aspects of bone disease are available by calling the toll-free number or downloading from the web site.

Osteoporosis Society of Canada
33 Laird Drive
Toronto, Ontario M4G 3S9 Canada
In Canada, (800) 463-6842
(416) 696-2663                    FAX (416) 696-2673

Provides public and professional education materials. Free publications list includes brochures in both English and French. Osteoporosis and Menopause Information Line, (800) 463-6842, provides individual counseling and recorded messages. Publishes semi-annual "Bulletin for Physicians" and "OsteoBlast" for contributors.

Women's Health Initiative (WHI)
Office of Disease Prevention, Office of the Director
National Institutes of Health
Federal Building, Room 6C12
7550 Wisconsin Avenue
Bethesda, MD 20892-9112
(301) 402-2900                    http://www.nih.gov/od/odp/whi/

This major women's health research project is examining the effects of estrogen replacement therapy (ERT) and calcium and vitamin D supplements on prevention of osteoporotic fractures. Women age 50 to 79 who wish to enroll should call (800) 549-6636.

Age Page: Preventing Falls and Fractures
National Institute on Aging (NIA)
NIA Information Center
Box 8057
Gaithersburg, MD 20898-8057
(800) 222-2225                          (301) 587-2528
e-mail: niainfo@access.digex.net

This pamphlet suggests ways in which elders can modify everyday activities and adapt the environment.  Large print.  Free

Arthritis, Rheumatic Diseases, and Related Disorders
National Arthritis and Musculoskeletal and Skin Diseases Information Clearinghouse
1 AMS Circle
Bethesda, MD 20892-3675
(301) 495-4484                    (301) 565-2966 (TT)                    FAX (301) 587-4352

This 1993 Special Report provides an overview of the research activities sponsored by the National Institutes of Health, including research on osteoporosis.  Free

Boning Up on Osteoporosis
National Osteoporosis Foundation (NOF)
1150 17th Street, NW, Suite 500
Washington, DC 20036
(800) 223-9994                    (202) 223-2226                    FAX (202) 223-2237
http://www.nof.org

This booklet includes information on the risk factors for osteoporosis, accident prevention, and posture and muscle strengthening exercises.  Members, free; nonmembers, $3.00.

Building Better Bones: A Guide to Active Living
Osteoporosis Society of Canada
33 Laird Drive
Toronto, Ontario M4G 3S9 Canada
In Canada, (800) 463-6842
(416) 696-2663                    FAX (416) 696-2673

This booklet describes the risk factors associated with osteoporosis, the role of nutrition and exercise in preventing osteoporosis, and hormone therapy.  Available in English and French.  $.50 (Canadian funds)

Facts About Osteoporosis, Arthritis, and Osteoarthritis
National Osteoporosis Foundation (NOF)
1150 17th Street, NW, Suite 500
Washington, DC 20036
(800) 223-9994                    (202) 223-2226                    FAX (202) 223-2237
http://www.nof.org

This booklet describes the difference between osteoporosis and two common types of arthritis. Discusses how treatment for arthritis may affect the development of osteoporosis.  Free

Home Safety Checklist for Older Consumers
U.S. Consumer Product Safety Commission
Washington, DC  20207
(800) 638-2772

Provides information on simple, inexpensive repairs and safety recommendations.  Available in English and Spanish.  Free

Instructional Video Tapes for Patients with Osteoporosis
Osteoporosis Society of Canada
33 Laird Drive
Toronto, Ontario M4G 3S9 Canada
In Canada, (800) 463-6842          (416) 696-2817                    FAX (416) 696-2673

Series of four videotapes: "Osteoporosis: What Is It?," "Exercise for Osteoporosis," "Nutrition for Osteoporosis," and "Coping with Osteoporosis."  Available in English and French.  $35.00 each, Canadian funds.

Living with Osteoporosis
National Osteoporosis Foundation (NOF)
1150 17th Street, NW, Suite 500
Washington, DC 20036
(800) 223-9994                    (202) 223-2226                    FAX (202) 223-2237
http://www.nof.org

This booklet provides tips for everyday living with osteoporosis.  Includes recommendations for preventing falls and making every room in the home safe.  Free

Medications and Bone Loss
National Osteoporosis Foundation (NOF)
1150 17th Street, NW, Suite 500
Washington, DC 20036
(800) 223-9994                    (202) 223-2226                    FAX (202) 223-2237
http://www.nof.org

This booklet discusses how medications such as steroids, taken for other medical conditions, may increase the risk of developing osteoporosis.  Free

The Older Person's Guide to Osteoporosis
National Osteoporosis Foundation (NOF)
1150 17th Street, NW, Suite 500
Washington, DC 20036
(800) 223-9994     (202) 223-2226     FAX (202) 223-2237
http://www.nof.org

This booklet provides a basic overview of the condition.  Free

Osteoporosis
Arthritis Foundation
1314 Spring Street, NW
Atlanta, GA 30309
(800) 283-7800     (404) 872-7100     FAX (404) 872-0457
http://www@arthritis.org

This booklet provides information about causes, symptoms, diagnosis, and treatment of osteoporosis.
Includes home safety check list.  Free

Osteoporosis
National Arthritis and Musculoskeletal and Skin Diseases Information Clearinghouse
1 AMS Circle
Bethesda, MD 20892-3675
(301) 495-4484     (301) 565-2966 (TT)    FAX (301) 587-4352

This information packet contains medical articles, patient information, fact sheets, and a glossary.
Free

Osteoporosis: A Woman's Guide
National Osteoporosis Foundation (NOF)
1150 17th Street, NW, Suite 500
Washington, DC 20036
(800) 223-9994     (202) 223-2226     FAX (202) 223-2237
http://www.nof.org

This brochure provides general information about osteoporosis.  Available in standard print and large
print.  Free

Osteoporosis: Basic Exercise Program
Osteoporosis Society of Canada
33 Laird Drive
Toronto, Ontario M4G 3S9 Canada
In Canada, (800) 463-6842   (416) 696-2663     FAX (416) 696-2673

This videotape provides instruction in basic exercises for individuals at various stages of osteoporosis.
64 minutes.  $39.95, Canadian funds.

The Osteoporosis Handbook
by Sydney Lou Bonnick
Taylor Publishing Company
1550 West Mockingbird Lane
Dallas, TX 75235
(800) 677-2800                    FAX (214) 819-8580

Written by a physician, this book describes the diagnosis and treatment of osteoporosis. Includes chapters on exercising to prevent osteoporosis as well as exercises for women with the condition. $14.95 plus $3.00 shipping and handling.

Osteoporosis: How to Make Your Bones Last a Lifetime
by Wanda S. Lyon and Cynthia E. Sutton
Contemporary Books
2 Prudential Plaza, Suite 1200
Chicago, IL 60601
(800) 621-1918                    (312) 540-4500                    FAX (312) 540-4687
Order FAX (800) 998-3103

This book provides information on the condition as well as screening, diagnosis, and treatment. Includes recipes rich in calcium, a glossary, and suggestions for preventing falls and other accidents. $10.99 plus 10% shipping and handling.

Osteoporosis: Progress and Prevention
Films for the Humanities & Sciences
PO Box 2053
Princeton, NJ 08543-2053
(800) 257-5126                    FAX (609) 275-3767

This videotape describes diagnosis and screening techniques as well as treatment. Discusses the risk factors for osteoporosis and its relationship to menopause and estrogen. $99.00 plus $5.75 shipping and handling.

Preventing Osteoporosis
American College of Obstetricians and Gynecologists
409 12th Street, SW
Washington, DC 20024-2188
(202) 638-5577                    http://www.acog.com

This brochure describes the condition, risk factors, and prevention. Discusses hormone replacement therapy, and includes a chart of foods containing calcium. Free

Stand UP to Osteoporosis
National Osteoporosis Foundation (NOF)
1150 17th Street, NW, Suite 500
Washington, DC 20036
(800) 223-9994                    (202) 223-2226                    FAX (202) 223-2237
http://www.nof.org

This brochure describes the condition, risk factors, preventive measures, diagnosis, and treatment. Free

Strategies for People with Osteoporosis
National Osteoporosis Foundation (NOF)
1150 17th Street, NW, Suite 500
Washington, DC 20036
(800) 223-9994                    (202) 223-2226              FAX (202) 223-2237
http://www.nof.org

This packet of articles offers suggestions for coping with osteoporosis, including what to do after diagnosis, recovery from fractures, and safety in the home.  $8.00

Talking with Your Doctor about Osteoporosis
National Osteoporosis Foundation (NOF)
1150 17th Street, NW, Suite 500
Washington, DC 20036
(800) 223-9994                    (202) 223-2226              FAX (202) 223-2237

This booklet lists questions women of all ages should ask their physicians about preventing osteoporosis, including topics such as exercise, diet, and lifestyle.  Available in standard print and large print.  Free

# Chapter 10

# *SPINAL CORD INJURY*

Injury to the spinal cord is a traumatic physical injury as well as a serious psychological injury. Because the spinal cord is responsible for transmitting the brain's electrical impulses that control other organs of the body, an injury to the spinal cord affects many of the body's systems. Required modifications of life style may be extreme, depending upon the severity of the injury. When a spinal cord injury occurs in a woman who is expecting to have a family or who already has young children, her plans for the future may seem to go awry. Although the effects of the injury may be overwhelming at first, rehabilitation opportunities and the development of a wide variety of special assistive devices have enabled thousands of individuals with spinal cord injuries to live productive lives and to continue to participate in many recreational activities, albeit in modified forms.

It has been estimated that there are about 200,000 living Americans who have experienced spinal cord injuries, the majority of whom were injured during or after World War II. Prior to World War II and the development of penicillin and sulfa drugs that prevent death from urinary tract infections, it was unusual for those who had a spinal cord injury to survive (DeVivo et al.: 1987). Today, due to the development of these drugs and improved emergency medical care at the scene of accidents, the vast majority of individuals with spinal cord injuries live for many years.

Studies of patients admitted to the Model Spinal Cord Injury Care Systems (Stover: 1994) have yielded demographic characteristics about the population. About one-fifth (19.2%) of individuals with spinal cord injuries are females; the average age at onset is 33.4 years. Automobile accidents account for 38.1% of all spinal cord injuries. Since 1990, violence as a cause of spinal cord injury has increased to 25.1%; domestic violence against women has recently been recognized as a growing cause of spinal cord injury. A study of women with spinal cord injuries in one metropolitan area found that 28% had experienced violence that caused their injuries (White et al.: 1996). Sports accidents are a major cause of spinal cord injuries among the younger population, while falls are a major cause among the older population. Tumors and diseases such as poliomyelitis, arthritis, spina bifida, and multiple sclerosis may also cause spinal cord injuries.

A recent study (DeVivo et al.: 1992) investigated the characteristics of men and women who had received treatment for spinal cord injury at six federally supported model treatment centers between 1973 and 1986. The study found several significant differences between the population who had been injured in the period 1973-77 and those who had been injured in the period 1984-86; the mean age at the time of injury increased over time as did the proportion of individuals who were not white and the proportion with quadriplegia. Although the mean length of stays in hospitals for rehabilitation decreased, the cost of the rehabilitation increased. For those who entered the centers within the first 24 hours of injury, the probability of dying in the first two years following injury decreased by two-thirds. While virtually all of the subjects were discharged to live in the community during the entire study period, only a small percentage of the subjects were employed two years post-injury, ranging from a low of 12.5% in the 1978-80 period to a high of 14.7% for those who had been injured from 1984-86. While a substantial proportion were students and small proportions were either homemakers or retired two years post-injury, over half of the subjects were unemployed throughout the study period.

Women with spinal cord injuries comprise an underemployed group. Bonwich (1985) found that 31 of 36 respondents had worked prior to their injury, but at the time of her interviews only eight of the 36 were working full-time. This low rate of employment is consistent with other studies (for example, DeVivo et al.: 1992). Charlifue and colleagues (1992) found that level of impairment was significantly related to rates of employment; while 59% of women with incomplete paraplegia held jobs, only 18% of those with complete quadriplegia held jobs. Women with higher levels of education are more likely to be employed following spinal cord injury, because their work is usually sedentary and requires little physical activity.

## THE SPINAL CORD

The spine has 33 bony, hollow, interlocking vertebrae including seven cervical or neck vertebrae, 12 thoracic or high back vertebrae, five lumbar or low back vertebrae, five sacral vertebrae near the base of the spine, and four coccygeal vertebrae fused to form the coccyx. The spinal cord, consisting of a narrow bundle of nerve cells and fibers, runs from the base of the brain through the hollow structure of the vertebrae. The brain's communication with the rest of the body is carried out through these nerve fibers.

Paralysis, the loss or impairment of motor function, occurs below the site of the injury or fracture. Not all injuries are complete, meaning that sometimes the individual may retain some sensation or movement below the site of the injury. *Paraplegia*, or paralysis of the legs and often the lower part of the body, occurs when the spinal cord is injured at the thoracic, lumbar, or sacral level of the spine. When injuries are complete, individuals also lose their sense of touch, pain, and temperature in the affected region.

*Quadriplegia* (or tetraplegia) is paralysis of all four limbs and the part of the body beneath the site of the spinal cord injury. Quadriplegia occurs when the injury to the spinal cord is at the level of the cervical vertebrae or the neck region. The lower the lesion within the cervical area, the greater amount of function that remains. Some individuals with cervical spinal cord injuries retain some function of the shoulders, biceps, upper arms, and the wrists. In general, the higher the site of the injury, the less function the individual retains. Individuals whose injuries are complete and at the chin level require respirators in order to breathe. These individuals require assistance with their everyday activities, although the use of mouthsticks and sip-and-puff mechanisms enables them to operate wheelchairs, computers, and other devices (Trieschmann: 1988).

According to Young and his associates (1982), there is a higher prevalence of quadriplegia (53%) than paraplegia (47%), but the injuries are more likely to be complete in paraplegia (60%) than quadriplegia (52%).

## TREATMENT AND COMPLICATIONS OF SPINAL CORD INJURY

Acute medical care following an accident that has caused spinal cord injury includes x-rays, possible treatment for shock, and immobilization of the patient. Patients are often placed in a Stryker frame, which is used to immobilize the spine and prevent further injury. A catheter to control bladder function is inserted, and urine output is monitored. In some cases, surgery may be performed to stabilize or fuse the spine, free nerve roots, or remove bony fragments. Immediately following the injury, swelling and bruising near the site of the fracture may be present, preventing the determination of the extent of neurological damage (Trieschmann: 1988). Patients are positioned and turned frequently in an effort to prevent pressure sores (see below). Other injuries that often accompany spinal cord injuries, such as fractures and lung injuries, must also be treated. Pain may also be a major problem in the first weeks following injury.

Preliminary studies on the use of drugs immediately following spinal cord injury have found some positive benefits. Administration of methylprednisolone within eight hours following the injury resulted in the recovery of an average of 20% of the motor and sensory function lost (Hingley: 1993).

Although treatments have been developed for many of the complications of spinal cord injury, it is still necessary to constantly be aware of the development of these complications and to take measures to prevent them. ***Pressure sores*** or ***decubitus ulcers*** are lesions on the skin that usually occur over a bony surface and result from lack of motion. Because the individual may have no sensation at the site where the sores begin to develop, they may become deep before they are discovered. In an effort to prevent pressure sores, individuals who are confined to bed immediately following the injury should be moved frequently and great attention should be paid to cleansing the skin regularly. Special flotation pads and sheepskins are sometimes used to relieve pressure and distribute body weight. Because of their restricted mobility, individuals with spinal cord injuries must take precautions to prevent pressure sores for the rest of their lives.

Despite the loss of sensation to temperature and touch below the site of the lesion, ***pain*** and unusual sensations may be a problem for people with spinal cord injuries. According to Trieschmann (1988), until recently it was assumed that pain was not a problem, and little attention was paid to the subject. However, Trieschmann states that many individuals experience a tingling or pins and needles sensation as well as other types of pain, such as shooting or burning sensations.

***Transcutaneous electric nerve stimulation*** (TENS) is a treatment method for pain in which low level electric impulses are delivered to nerve endings under the skin near the source of pain. It is not known why TENS should be effective in relieving pain or if it is really effective. Research is currently underway to gain a better understanding of the way in which this procedure works.

***Loss of bladder and bowel control*** is another complication of spinal cord injury. Those individuals who have indwelling catheters are prone to develop bladder infections. When the extent of nerve damage permits, it is preferable to have the individual learn how to control her bladder through an individualized training program. Similarly, programs for bowel control enable the individual to empty the bowel on a regular schedule, thereby avoiding gastrointestinal complications such as distention and impaction. Attention to diet and the use of rectal suppositories may also contribute to control of bowel movements.

***Spasticity*** (involuntary jerky motions) is common in individuals with spinal cord injuries. These spasms are caused by random stimulation of the nerves leading to the muscles. Severe spasms may interfere with some activity and in some cases may be strong enough to throw the individual from the bed or chair.

***Functional electrical stimulation*** (FES) is an experimental method that uses electrical stimulation to evoke skeletal muscle responses in areas that do not function normally because injury or disease has cut off the pathway for central nervous system communication from the brain. A functional electrical stimulation system consists of a control unit, a stimulator unit, and electrodes. In some instances, the goal of functional electrical stimulation is to restore movement or function and in other cases to strengthen muscles. A study by Petrofsky (1992) found that subjects with spinal cord injuries who participated in a two year experiment using functional electrical stimulation to exercise muscles had a reduction in the incidence of pressure sores and urinary tract infections. Another experiment (Granat et al.: 1992) that used functional electrical stimulation to restore movement in six subjects with incomplete spinal cord injury found that all subjects were able to stand and walk using an FES system, but half of the subjects found that the system was not practical for their lifestyles.

As more individuals with spinal cord injuries survive longer, they are also experiencing the normal physiological processes that accompany aging. There is little information on how these processes affect people with spinal cord injuries who have been disabled for many years. The effects of menopause on women with spinal cord injuries are unknown. However, preliminary indications are that physiological changes associated with aging have a greater impact on people with spinal cord injuries. Menter (1990) calls this phase "decline," noting that there is a decrease in muscle strength, range of motion, and respiratory and cardiovascular capacity and an increase in the breakdown of the skin.

The National Institute of Neurological Disorders and Stroke (see "ORGANIZATIONS" section below) is currently funding innovative research that may someday enable clinicians to restore function to those who have experienced spinal cord injury. Some promising innovations include treatment with steroids, promoting new growth in damaged nerves, and using electronic prostheses to carry out the functions previously achieved by the damaged nerves.

## SEXUAL FUNCTIONING

Spinal cord injury may affect sexual functioning in both men and women, although the effects are greater for men. Women often temporarily stop menstruating upon injury, but most will resume menstruating within six months and may conceive and bear children. Rehabilitation programs for people with spinal cord injuries should include counseling in the area of sexual functioning; however, a recent study found that only 37% of the women with spinal cord injuries had received information related to sexual functioning compared to 66% of the men with spinal cord injuries (White et al.: 1994). Many of the counseling programs that do exist are oriented toward male sexuality, and little research has been done on female sexuality following spinal cord injury. Counseling by trained professionals can help alleviate some of the fears and anxieties that women hold about their sexuality. Suggestions for alternative positions and techniques to use during sexual relations can be invaluable, especially if the woman's partner is included in the discussion.

The lack of mobility caused by spinal cord injury changes the role that women play in sexual relationships. Individuals who have spinal cord injuries lose sensation in the parts of their bodies that are below the lesion in their spinal cord; they may derive pleasure through stimulation of parts of the body above the injury. The ability to produce adequate lubrication and to feel sensation in the genital area varies, although little laboratory research exists on these subjects. Those women who do not produce adequate vaginal lubrication are advised to use commercial, water soluble lubricants.

Self-reports from women who have experienced spinal cord injuries suggest that many are able to achieve satisfying sexual relationships. One recent study of 25 women with spinal cord injuries reported that 44% were able to achieve orgasm (Sipski and Alexander: 1993). The same study found that the favorite sexual activities of women with spinal cord injuries were kissing, hugging, and touching, whereas intercourse was the favorite activity prior to their injury. A more recent study carried out by the same laboratory (Sipski et al.: 1995) found that over half of the women with spinal cord injuries (52%) achieved orgasm compared to all of the women without spinal cord injuries. The study was not able to identify any characteristics that could predict whether women with spinal cord injuries would achieve orgasm. A study by Charlifue and colleagues (1992) reported that 69% of the subjects were satisfied with their sex life following spinal cord injury, and about half said that they were capable of achieving orgasm. However, the women reported that sexual activity was not as important to them as it was before their injury. A study of 15 women with spinal cord injuries found that the use of fantasy resulted in increased sexual pleasure (Berard: 1989). Those women who did not fantasize and in fact had abandoned their sexuality were less likely to have accepted their disability. Women who have recently experienced spinal cord injuries may find it difficult to resume a sexual relationship or to begin a relationship with a new partner. As in all sexual relationships, good communication facilitates the process. When women feel comfortable talking to their partners, they can discuss their preferences and ways to experiment with new positions and techniques that were not used prior to their injuries.

Most women with spinal cord injuries are sexually active; one recent study found that 65% had had sexual intercourse within the year prior to the study. However, these women still express a number of concerns related to their sexual relationships. The most common concerns expressed by these women are fear of urinary and bowel accidents, not satisfying a partner, and feeling sexually unattractive (White et al.: 1994).

Fear of bladder and bowel incontinence during sexual relations may result in avoidance of sexual relations. It is not necessary for women with indwelling catheters to remove them during sex, although some may feel more comfortable doing so. Women who are on regular bowel programs are advised to empty their bowel prior to sexual activity to avoid the fear of bowel accidents.

In cases where attendant care is necessary (usually in cases of quadriplegia), the partner often becomes a caretaker by default when financial resources do not permit hiring an attendant. Yet some women have difficulty conceiving of a sexual relationship if their partners assist with their bladder and bowel control (Friedman Becker: 1978). For other women, their partner's role as personal attendant is viewed as normal and does not create problems in the area of sexual relationships. In those instances where a paid personal attendant helps the woman with her bodily functions, it is often necessary for the attendant to prepare and position the woman for sexual intercourse. Since being involved in another person's intimate affairs may cause embarrassment or tension, an open discussion between the attendant and the partners may prove useful.

## FAMILY PLANNING, PREGNANCY, AND CHILDREARING

Spinal cord injury does not affect a woman's fertility, and in most instances women can deliver their babies vaginally. Recent medical literature suggests that most women with spinal cord injuries who do become pregnant have excellent outcomes for both themselves and their babies (Baker and Cardenas: 1996). One study found that over a third of women with spinal cord injuries decided not to have children, and most of these women attributed their decision to the injury (Charlifue et al.: 1992). Methods of contraception are somewhat limited for women with spinal cord injuries. Limited mobility often prevents the placement of a diaphragm. Birth control pills may increase the risk of blood clots, which are already a higher probability for women with spinal cord injuries because of their inactivity. A relatively new form of birth control, Norplant, prevents ovulation for up to five years through the implantation of synthetic progesterone. However, removal of the implant has caused both scarring and pain in some women. Some women who have definitely decided not to have children choose to have tubal ligation, a procedure that is sometimes reversible.

During pregnancy, women may be more likely to develop decubitus ulcers due to weight gain, and transfers become more difficult toward the latter part of the term. Most women with spinal cord injuries do develop urinary tract infections during pregnancy, in part due to indwelling catheters. Avoidance of indwelling catheters and the use of antibiotics may help to prevent this condition (Baker and Cardenas: 1996).

The ability of women to feel labor pains varies with the level of the lesion. It has been recommended that women with spinal cord injuries be hospitalized in preparation for labor as soon as they begin to dilate or at the thirty-second week of gestation (Patel: 1989). A condition called autonomic dysreflexia, in which drastic changes occur in body temperature, heart rate, and blood pressure, is a risk during labor for women with spinal cord injuries, especially when the lesion is at or above the sixth thoracic vertebra (Broderson: 1990; Patel: 1989). For this reason, women with spinal cord injuries should plan to deliver their babies in hospitals equipped to handle this type of condition.

The types of devices and adaptations that are necessary for child care vary with the woman's level of injury, her home environment, and the amount of assistance she receives from family members and paid help. Possible options include special trays that attach to wheelchairs and hold the baby (Through the Looking Glass: 1994). Some women with spinal cord injuries find that the most difficult stage of childrearing is when babies begin to crawl around the home; at this stage it is difficult for the mothers to control their child's actions and safety. However, as children learn to respond to verbal requests made by the mother, the mother's lack of mobility becomes less of an issue. Women with spinal cord injuries have noted that their children quickly learn to respond to verbal discipline, become involved in household activities, and develop independence at an early age. As children begin socializing with other children in the neighborhood and at school, they must learn to respond effectively to the taunts they may receive about their mother's condition. Some mothers may wish to visit their children's classrooms to explain their condition and to answer questions, so that classmates feel more comfortable and interested in visiting their home.

## PSYCHOLOGICAL ASPECTS OF SPINAL CORD INJURY

Women who experience spinal cord injuries as a result of an accident have had no preparation for life with a disability. In an instant, they have changed from able-bodied women into women with severe physical limitations. The suddenness with which this change takes place and the wide ranging effects are likely to cause great anguish to the individuals as well as to their families and friends. The more severe the disability, the greater the loss of independence. For many women, these circumstances result in a loss of self-esteem and fear of re-entering the larger community. It is essential that women with spinal cord injuries receive help with their emotional adjustment, either in the form of individual or group counseling from professionals or through self-help groups and role models of other women who have adjusted successfully to spinal cord injuries.

Because most of the individuals who experience spinal cord injuries are males, women who have spinal cord injuries may feel isolated and without accessible peers or role models. They may need counseling about sexual functioning; the physical aspects of becoming pregnant; handling the responsibilities of motherhood; and other physical and emotional issues that affect women. Yet it is not unusual for a woman to be the only woman in a spinal cord injury unit or one of two or three women (Scheele: 1988). In a vulnerable position to start with, these women may feel uncomfortable asking the questions they have when health care and rehabilitation professionals have oriented their services to men. Obtaining support and counsel from other women who have successfully adjusted to spinal cord injuries may prove enormously beneficial to recently injured women.

Because the traditional role of women in society has been characterized by passivity and dependence, some observers have suggested that women will adjust better to spinal cord injuries than men, as spinal cord injuries result in dependence. The women's movement has expanded women's roles in society, with more women independent both financially and emotionally. Further, some women have experienced spinal cord injuries as a result of their physical activity, such as horseback riding or other athletic activities. These women must adjust to great modifications in everyday activities and loss of leisure activities that they valued.

A spinal cord injury often places a woman's self-esteem in jeopardy, as she questions her physical attractiveness and her ability to attract and satisfy a sexual partner. While men are judged based on power, wealth, career, and physical accomplishments, women are judged largely on their physical attractiveness.

In contrast to observers such as Trieschmann (1988) who contend that adjustment to spinal cord injury is more difficult for women than for men, Bonwich (1985) has noted that for some women with spinal cord injuries, self-esteem actually increases through what she refers to as "role gain." No longer tied down to traditional norms of what is expected of women, these women master a new role which is quite demanding and live up to their potential.

Some women may never lose the anger or guilt they feel about the circumstances surrounding the accident that caused the injury. In the period immediately following the accident, they may feel overpowered by the many professionals who have begun to make major decisions for them. In some cases, the accidents that caused spinal cord injuries involved the use of alcohol while driving. These factors, combined with inadequate counseling and the inability to cope with the effects of the injury, result in the abuse of alcohol or other drugs. Bozzacco (1990) suggests that all patients in rehabilitation units be assessed for their vulnerability to alcohol and drug abuse. She further suggests that patients become part of the decision-making process for their own treatment and rehabilitation plans as soon as possible and that alcohol and drug treatment programs be an integral part of rehabilitation.

The need to modify the activities of everyday living as well as the physical environment; the impairment of sexual functioning; and the financial aspects of living with spinal cord injury may place a great strain on marital and family relationships. In some instances, partners of women with spinal cord injuries deny that she has experienced an enormous change and that there will be a great impact on their relationship and roles (Friedman Becker: 1978). For this reason, it is helpful to include the partner in the rehabilitation and counseling program.

Although Young and his associates (1982) found that four years after spinal cord injury, nearly the same percentage of females (17%) and males (16%) were divorced, another study found that females were far more likely than males to be divorced. Brown and Giesy (1986) found that 40.6% of the females they studied were divorced/separated/widowed versus 15.9% for the general population. For males the corresponding figures were 18.1% and 9.3%. Similarly, they found that 26.1% of the females were married compared to 65.2% in the general population; 40.7% of the males were married compared to 62.6% in the general population. These findings suggest that spinal cord injuries are more difficult for women than for men in the area of marital relationships, despite the fact that women's sexual functioning is less impaired than men's.

Those women with severe injuries often require the help of a paid personal attendant to perform tasks related to bodily function and cleanliness. Although there is some government assistance to pay for these services, in most instances family members carry out these tasks. It is also common for family members in this role to feel both overburdened and guilty. Social workers should work with the family to arrange for respite care, financial assistance, and other services that can remediate the situation.

## PROFESSIONAL SERVICE PROVIDERS

In most cases, the physician in charge serves as the case manager or coordinator for the person with spinal cord injury. The physician in charge may be a *physiatrist* (a specialist trained in rehabilitation medicine); an *orthopedist* (a specialist in treatment of the skeletal system); or a *neurologist* or *neurosurgeon* (a specialist in disorders of the nervous system). All of these physicians receive training in treatment of spinal cord injuries. Also on the multidisciplinary team are *urologists*, who specialize in treatment of kidneys, the bladder, the ureter, and the urethra. *Obstetricians/gynecologists* may also play an important role in helping women with spinal cord injuries to deliver their babies safely; these physicians should work in conjunction with others who specialize in the care and rehabilitation of women with spinal cord injuries.

*Rehabilitation nurses* receive special training available at schools throughout the country and may receive certification in this specialty after working two years in a rehabilitation setting (Livingston: 1991). They work closely with the physicians and in some instances may serve as case managers. In inpatient settings, rehabilitation nurses work with other health care and rehabilitation professionals to develop and implement medical and rehabilitation plans for patients. They may act as consultants in planning for discharge and may evaluate the individual's home to ensure that appropriate environmental modifications have been made. They are often the professionals in charge of following up on the individual's needs after discharge from the rehabilitation unit.

*Orthotists* specialize in the design of braces and other devices that help with mobility, support, and prevention of further injury. They also fit the devices and provide instruction in their use. *Rehabilitation engineers* specialize in the design of devices that enable people with disabilities to function at their maximum level of independence. Their research includes the development of robotic devices and other computer driven devices that serve as substitutes for the function that was lost as a result of injury or disease. In some instances, they may consult on individual cases to adapt wheelchairs or other devices for specific needs.

*Physical therapists* design exercise programs to maintain and strengthen residual motor function. They also teach transfer skills to and from the bed and how to use wheelchairs and orthotic devices, such as canes, braces, and walkers. They develop exercise programs to help individuals who are able to use crutches to build up muscles in their arms and shoulders.

· *Occupational therapists* teach individuals with spinal cord injuries how to re-learn the activities of daily living. Included are eating, dressing, grooming, and the use of "high tech" devices that contribute to increased independence. After assessing a woman's home environment, family situation, and place of employment, the occupational therapist may recommend specially adapted equipment or environmental adaptations to enable her to continue with her activities.

*Psychologists* provide individual or group counseling to women with spinal cord injuries and to their family members. They may also provide special help in the area of sexual functioning. *Social workers* help to make the arrangements that enable individuals to return to the community. They also ensure that individuals with spinal cord injuries receive the financial assistance that they are entitled to. Social workers may also provide counseling for women and their families. In some instances, social workers or psychologists have developed group counseling or peer support groups especially for women with spinal cord injuries.

## WHERE TO FIND SERVICES

The federal government sponsors the "Model System of Spinal Cord Injury Care" in order to provide coordinated comprehensive care and to conduct research related to spinal cord injury. Administered by the National Institute on Disability and Rehabilitation Research (NIDRR) within the U.S. Department of Education, this model system encompasses treatment centers throughout the country that participate in research and data collection efforts. The major components of the model system include early access to care through rapid, effective transportation; an acute level one traumatology setting; a comprehensive acute rehabilitation program; psychosocial and vocational services that begin in the hospital and continue through discharge; and follow-up to ascertain that medical and psychosocial needs are met once patients have re-entered the community (Thomas: 1990).

Another federal system that offers special treatment for individuals with spinal cord injuries is the U.S. Department of Veteran Affairs (VA). Spinal cord units are located at a number of VA Medical Centers across the country. The National Institutes of Health also funds model research and treatment centers at several facilities.

Many rehabilitation hospitals have spinal cord injury units. The advantage of obtaining treatment in these settings is that other patients serve as role models. Some acute care hospitals also have rehabilitation units, and outpatient rehabilitation facilities offer services to people with spinal cord injuries. Many long term care facilities provide services to people with spinal cord injuries. The Commission on Accreditation of Rehabilitation Facilities (CARF) provides accreditation for these facilities (see "ORGANIZATIONS" section below). Independent living centers offer services and referrals to people with spinal cord injuries.

## MODIFICATIONS IN EVERYDAY LIVING

In order to remain living in the community, many women with spinal cord injuries, especially those with quadriplegia, require personal attendant services (PAS). Personal attendant services may be provided by a family member, friend, or a person specifically employed for this purpose. Personal attendants perform tasks that enable the woman with a disability to carry out her activities of daily living. A variety of health care providers have observed that personal attendant services contribute not only to the improved physical well-being of individuals with spinal cord injuries and other disabilities, but also to their mental well-being (Nosek: 1993).

The major source of funding for the employment of personal attendants is Medicaid, although other state, local, and federal programs as well as private agencies often contribute. According to Nosek (19 91), most individuals with disabilities rely on family members and have had no contacts with formal programs that provide personal attendants. Furthermore, those interested in hiring personal attendants often have difficulty locating qualified individuals. A number of consumer advocacy organizations, research organizations, and the federal government are paying increased attention to the issue of personal attendant services in an attempt to improve the provision of these services.

Most women with spinal cord injuries use wheelchairs for mobility. A wide variety of wheelchairs designed for different purposes and different types of impairments is available. Women whose injury prohibits them from using manually operated wheelchairs may use battery operated wheelchairs. Sip-and-puff controls, tubes that respond to changes in pressure caused by inhaling and exhaling, enable women with more severe impairments to control the movement of their wheelchairs. Wheelchairs are prescribed by physicians and must accommodate the individual's body size, disability, and functional criteria.

Women whose injury has resulted in paraplegia sometimes use braces as an alternative to wheelchairs. One study (Heinemann et al.: 1987) found that only about a quarter of those individuals who had braces continued to use them, while the remainder preferred using wheelchairs. Those who continued to use braces were less likely to have complete lesions than those who stopped using braces. Those who stopped using braces said that they preferred wheelchairs because they were safer, required less energy, and were less likely to fail.

Modification of the home environment requires the installation of ramps; wide doorways with doors that open easily; the removal of thresholds between rooms; and lifts for getting from one level of the home to the other. The kitchen should have accessible appliances, shelves, and working space, and pulls and knobs that are easy to use. The bathroom should be large enough to accommodate a wheelchair; the sink must be at an accessible level; showers should be the roll-in variety with grab bars; and toilets should have grab bars.

Many individuals with paraplegia learn to drive with special hand controls, locks, steering mechanisms, and wheelchair lifts. Major automobile manufacturers offer special programs to purchase adapted vehicles with special controls and wheelchair lifts (see Chapter 2, "ORGANIZATIONS," page 85).

Special feeding devices are available for individuals with quadriplegia who do not have the use of their upper limbs. Devices may be installed that move people around a room. Use of these specialized devices increases the independence of individuals with quadriplegia.

References

Baker, Emily R. and Diana D. Cardenas
1996 "Pregnancy in Spinal Cord Injured Women" Archives of Physical Medicine and Rehabilitation 77(May):501-507

Berard, E. J. J.
1989 "The Sexuality of Spinal Cord Injured Women: Physiology and Pathophysiology. A Review" Paraplegia 27: 99-112

Bonwich, Emily
1985 "Sex Role Attitudes and Role Reorganization in Spinal Cord Injured Women" pp. 56-67 in Mary Jo Deegan and Nancy A. Brooks (eds.) Women and Disability: The Double Handicap New Brunswick, NJ: Transaction Inc.

Bozzacco, Victoria
1990 "Vulnerability and Alcohol and Substance Abuse in Spinal Cord Injury" Rehabilitation Nursing 15(Mar.-Apr.):2:70-72

Broderson, Linda C.
1990 "Motherhood, Pregnancy, and Spinal Cord Injury" Paraplegia News 44(October):110:50-53

Brown, Julia S. and Barbara Giesy
1986 "Marital Status of Persons with Spinal Cord Injury" Social Science and Medicine 23:3:313-322

Charlifue, S.W. et al.
1992 "Sexual Issues of Women With Spinal Cord Injuries" Paraplegia 30:192-199

DeVivo, Michael J. et al.
1992 "Trends in Spinal Cord Injury Demographics and Treatment Outcomes Between 1973 and 1986" Archives of Physical Medicine and Rehabilitation 73(May):424-430

1987 "Seven-Year Survival Following Spinal Cord Injury" Archives of Neurology 44(August):872-875

Friedman Becker, Elle
1978 Female Sexuality Following Spinal Cord Injury Bloomington, IL: Accent Special Publications

Granat, M. et al.
1992 "The Use of Functional Electrical Stimulation to Assist Gait in Patients with Incomplete Spinal Cord Injury" Disability and Rehabilitation 14(2):93-97

Heinemann, Allen W. et al.
1987 "Mobility for Persons with Spinal Cord Injury: An Evaluation of Two Systems" Archives of Physical Medicine and Rehabilitation 68(February):90-93

Hingley, Audrey T.
1993 "Spinal Cord Injuries: Science Meets Challenge" FDA Consumer July/August

Livingston, Carolyn
1991 "Opportunities in Rehabilitation Nursing" American Journal of Nursing 91 (Feb.):2:90-95

Menter, Robert R.
1990 "Aging and Spinal Cord Injury: Implications for Existing Model Systems and Future Federal, State, and Local Health Care Policy" pp. 72-80 in David F. Apple and Lesley M. Hudson (eds.) Spinal Cord Injury: The Model Atlanta, GA: Spinal Cord Injury Care System, Sheperd Center for the Treatment of Spinal Injuries

Nosek, Margaret A.

1993 "Personal Assistance: Its Effect on the Long-Term Health of a Rehabilitation Hospital Population" Archives of Physical Medicine and Rehabilitation 74(February):127-132

1991 "Personal Assistance Services: A Review of the Literature and Analysis of Policy Implications" Journal of Disability Policy Studies 2(2):1-17

Patel, Madhura V.

1989 "Management of Pregnancy in Women with Spinal Cord Injury and Traumatic Brain Injury" Sexuality Update 2(October):1:1-3

Petrofsky, Jerrold S.

1992 "Functional Electrical Stimulation, A Two-Year Study," Journal of Rehabilitation July/August/September 29-34

Scheele, Chris

1988 "Women and SCI Part 1: Overview" Paraplegia News March 41-43

Sipski, Marca L. and Craig J. Alexander

1993 "Sexual Activities, Response and Satisfaction in Women Pre- and Post-Spinal Cord Injury" Archives of Physical Medicine and Rehabilitation 74(October):1025-1029

Sipski, Marca L., Craig J. Alexander, and Raymond C. Rosen

1995 "Orgasm in Women with Spinal Cord Injuries: A Laboratory-Based Assessment" Archives of Physical Medicine and Rehabilitation 76(December):1097-1102

Stover, Samuel L.

1994 "Spinal Cord Injury: Knowns and Unknowns" Journal of the American Paraplegia Society 17(January):1:1-6

Thomas, J. Paul

1990 "Definition of the Model System of Spinal Cord Injury Care" pp. 7-9 in David F. Apple and Lesley M. Hudson (eds.) Spinal Cord Injury: The Model Atlanta, GA: Spinal Cord Injury Care System, Sheperd Center for the Treatment of Spinal Injuries

Through the Looking Glass

1994 "Adaptive Parenting Equipment" Parenting with a Disability 3(January)1:4

Trieschmann, Roberta B.

1988 Spinal Cord Injuries: Psychological, Social and Vocational Rehabilitation New York, NY: Demos Publications

White, Mary Joe et al.

1994 "A Comparison of the Sexual Concerns of Men and Women with Spinal Cord Injuries" Rehabilitation Nursing Research Summer:55-61

Young, John S. et al.

1982 Spinal Cord Injury Statistics Phoenix, AZ: Good Samaritan Medical Center

# ORGANIZATIONS

American Association of Spinal Cord Injury Nurses (AASCIN)
75-20 Astoria Boulevard
Jackson Heights, NY 11370
(718) 803-3782                    FAX (718) 803-0414

A professional membership organization that encourages and improves nursing care of individuals with spinal cord injuries and sponsors research. Publishes "SCI Nursing," quarterly. Membership, $75.00.

American Paralysis Association (APA)
500 Morris Avenue
Springfield, NJ 07081
(800) 225-0292                (201) 379-2690              FAX (201) 912-9433

Supports research to find a cure for paralysis caused by spinal cord injury and other central nervous system disorders. Publishes "Walking Tomorrow," a newsletter about the organization's activities, and "Progress in Research," a newsletter about spinal cord injury research. Various levels of membership dues.

American Paraplegia Society
75-20 Astoria Boulevard
Jackson Heights, NY 11370-1177
(718) 803-3782                  FAX (718) 803-0414

A professional membership organization for physicians, scientists, and allied health care professionals. Holds an annual meeting for the presentation of scientific research related to spinal cord injury. Membership, $100.00, includes quarterly journal, "Journal of the American Paraplegia Society."

American Rehabilitation Association
1910 Association Drive
Reston, VA 22091
(800) 368-3513                (703) 648-9300              FAX (703) 648-0346

A national membership organization of individuals and institutions that provide rehabilitation services. Conducts seminars, holds an annual meeting, and publishes a series of newsletters. Membership dues vary by income level.

American Spinal Injury Association (ASIA)
345 East Superior, Room 1436
Chicago, IL 60611
(312) 908-6207                FAX (312) 503-0869

A professional membership organization for health care providers dedicated to improving the care of individuals with spinal cord injury through research, education, and development of regional spinal cord injury care systems. Holds an annual meeting with presentation of scientific papers. Membership, physicians, $200.00; nonphysicians, $50.00; includes newsletter "ASIA Bulletin."

Center for Research on Women with Disabilities (CROWD)
Baylor College of Medicine
3440 Richmond Avenue, Suite B
Houston, TX 77046
(713) 960-0505 (V/TT)          FAX (713) 961-3555
e-mail: mnosek@bcm.tmc.edu     http://www.bcm.tmc.edu/crowd/

A federally funded center that conducts research and develops and distributes information on the health and independence of women with disabilities. Research areas include sexuality, relationships, general health, reproductive health, and abuse. Executive Summary of a four year "National Study on Women with Disabilities" is available; $20.00.

Commission on Accreditation of Rehabilitation Facilities (CARF)
4891 East Grant Road
Tucson, AZ 85712
(520) 325-1044 (V/TT)          FAX (520) 318-1129          http://www.carf.org

Conducts site evaluations and accredits organizations that provide rehabilitation. Publishes the "Directory of Accredited Organizations," $45.00 plus $5.50 shipping and handling.

Functional Electrical Stimulation Information Center
11000 Cedar Avenue
Cleveland, OH 44106-3052
(800) 666-2353                 (216) 231-3257 (V/TT)     FAX (216) 231-3258
e-mail: fes_info@po.cwru.edu   http://feswww.fes.cwru.edu

Affiliated with the Rehabilitation Engineering Center at Case Western Reserve University, the center provides information to consumers and professionals about functional electrical stimulation. Publishes quarterly newsletter, "FES Update," free. Free publications list.

International Foundation for Bowel Dysfunction
PO Box 17864
Milwaukee, WI 53217
(414) 964-1799

Provides information and support to individuals with functional gastrointestinal disorders, including incontinence due to spinal cord injury. Membership, $20.00, includes newsletter, "Participate."

Medical Rehabilitation Research and Training Center in Prevention and Treatment of Secondary Complications of Spinal Cord Injury
Spain Rehabilitation Center
University of Alabama at Birmingham
1717 Sixth Avenue South, Room 506
Birmingham, AL 35233
(205) 934-3283                 (205) 934-4642 (TT)       FAX (205) 975-4691
e-mail: Lindsey@sun.rehabm.uab.edu  http://www.sci.rehabm.uab.edu

A federally funded center that conducts research and holds educational conferences for individuals with spinal cord injuries and their families. Also holds training programs for professionals. The National Spinal Cord Injury Statistical Center collects data from spinal cord injury centers throughout the country. Produces a variety of audio-visual materials and books for professional care providers and consumers, as well as a series of information sheets. A list of articles documenting some of the center's research findings is also available. Their World Wide Web site contains a listing of organizations that provide services related to spinal cord injury as well as numerous links to other World Wide Web sites. A free newsletter, "Pushin' On," is published twice a year.

National Association for Continence (NAFC)
PO Box 8310
Spartanburg, SC 29305-8310
(800) 252-3337                    (864) 579-7900                    FAX (864) 579-7902
http://www.nafc.org

An information clearinghouse for consumers, family members, and medical professionals. Will answer individual questions if self-addressed stamped envelope is enclosed with letter. Membership, $15.00, includes a quarterly newsletter, "Quality Care," and a "Resource Guide: Products and Services for Continence" (nonmembers, $15.00). Free publications list.

National Institute of Neurological Disorders and Stroke (NINDS)
Building 31, Room 8A06
31 Center Drive, MSC 2540
Bethesda, MD 20892-2540
(800) 352-9424                    (301) 496-5751                    FAX (301) 402-2186
http://www.ninds.nih.gov

A federal agency that sponsors basic and clinical research to understand, prevent, and cure paralysis. Supports a national program of Spinal Cord Injury Research Centers located at Yale University in New Haven, CT; Ohio State University in Columbus, OH; University of Florida in Gainesville, FL; University of Miami in Miami, FL; Northwestern University in Chicago, IL; and New York University in New York, NY.

National Institute on Disability and Rehabilitation Research (NIDRR)
U.S. Department of Education
400 Maryland Avenue, SW
Washington, DC 20202
(202) 205-8134                    (202) 205-8198 (TT)                    FAX (202) 205-8515
http://www.ed.gov/offices/OSERS/NIDRR

A federal agency that supports research into various aspects of disability and rehabilitation, including demographic analyses, social science research, and the development of assistive devices. Supports a nationwide system of model spinal cord injury centers.

National Spinal Cord Injury Association (NSCIA)
8300 Colesville Road, Suite 551
Silver Spring, MD 20910
(800) 962-9629                    (301) 588-6959                 FAX (301) 588-9414
e-mail: NSCIA2@aol.com           http://www.spinalcord.org

A membership organization with chapters throughout the U.S. Disseminates information to people with spinal cord injuries and to their families; provides counseling; and advocates for the removal of barriers to independent living. Participates in the development of standards of care for regional spinal cord injury care. NSCIA will perform a customized database search; call for details. Holds annual meeting and educational seminars. Membership, individuals with a disability or family members, $25.00; allied health professionals, $50.00; attorneys or physicians, $100.00; organizations, $100.00; includes quarterly magazine, "Spinal Cord Injury Life" (nonmember price, $30.00), fact sheets, and discounts on other publications, medical products, and pharmaceutical supplies.

National Spinal Cord Injury Hotline
2200 Kernan Drive
Baltimore, MD 21207
(800) 526-3456                   FAX (410) 448-6628
e-mail: scihotline@aol.com       http://users.aol.com/scihotline

A 24 hour hotline that answers questions, solves individual problems, and makes referrals to professional service providers and peers with spinal cord injuries.

Paralyzed Veterans of America (PVA)
801 18th Street, NW
Washington, DC 20006
(800) 424-8200                   (800) 795-4327 (TT)            (202) 872-1300
FAX (202) 785-4452

A membership organization for veterans with spinal cord injury. Advocates and lobbies for the rights of paralyzed veterans and sponsors research. Publishes "Paraplegia News" and "Sports-N-Spokes" (see "PUBLICATIONS AND TAPES" section below). Membership dues are set by state chapters. The national office refers callers to the nearest chapter. The PVA Spinal Cord Injury Education and Training Foundation accepts applications to fund continuing education, post-professional specialty training, and patient/client and family education. The PVA Spinal Cord Research Foundation accepts applications to fund basic and clinical research, the design of assistive devices, and conferences that foster interaction among scientists and health care providers.

Rehabilitation Research and Training Center in Community Integration for Individuals with Spinal Cord Injury
Department of Physical Medicine and Rehabilitation
Baylor College of Medicine
One Baylor Plaza
Houston, TX 77030
(713) 960-1233

A federally funded center that conducts research and training on the health needs, psychological adjustment, and community integration of individuals with spinal cord injuries. Its training component, The Institute for Rehabilitation Research (TIRR) [1333 Moursund, Houston, TX 77030, (713) 797-5945], produces a variety of audiocassettes, videotapes, and publications for professionals, people with disabilities, and family members. Some materials have been translated into Spanish. TIRR will conduct special searches of its database on spinal cord injury (See National Database of Educational Resources on Spinal Cord Injury listed in "PUBLICATIONS AND TAPES" section below). Free publications list.

Rehabilitation Research and Training Center on Aging with Spinal Cord Injury
Craig Hospital
3425 South Clarkston
Englewood, CO 80110
(303) 789-8202                    FAX (303) 789-8441
http://www.Craig-Hospital.org/rehab

A federally funded center that studies the physiological and psychological effects of changes brought about by aging on individuals with spinal cord injuries. Produces consumer information brochures in English and Spanish and a semiannual newsletter, "Phases: SCI & Aging." Free

Rehabilitation Research and Training Center on Aging with Spinal Cord Injury
Rancho Los Amigos Medical Center
12481 Dahlia Street, Building 306
Downey, CA 90242
(310) 401-7402                    FAX (310) 401-7011

A federally funded center that trains service providers and consumers about spinal cord injury. Conducts research on the physiological and social aspects of aging with a spinal cord injury.

Simon Foundation for Continence
PO Box 815
Wilmette, IL 60091
(800) 237-4666                (708) 864-3913                FAX (708) 864-9758

Provides information and assistance to people who are incontinent. Organizes self-help groups. Membership, individuals, $15.00; professionals, $35.00; includes quarterly newsletter, "The Informer."

Vocational Rehabilitation Services
Veterans Benefits Administration
Department of Veterans Affairs (VA)
810 Vermont Avenue, NW
Washington, DC 20420
(202) 233-6496                (800) 827-1000 (connects with regional office)

Provides education, rehabilitation, and independent living services to veterans with service related disabilities through offices located in every state as well as regional centers, medical centers, and insurance centers. Medical services are provided at VA Medical Centers, Outpatient Clinics, Domiciliaries, and Nursing Homes.

Adaptive Parenting Equipment: Idea Book I
Through the Looking Glass
2198 Sixth Street, #100
Berkeley, CA 94710-2204
(800) 644-2666                    (510) 848-1112                    FAX (510) 848-4445
e-mail: tlg@lookingglass.org      http://www.lookingglass.org

A book that describes 50 products to help women with disabilities diaper, bathe, dress, feed, and play with their babies. Individuals, $10.00; organizations, $25.00.

Aerobics for Paraplegics
Aerobics for Quadriplegics
Disabled Sports, U.S.A.
451 Hungerford Drive, Suite 100
Rockville, Md 20850
(301) 217-0960                    (301) 217-0963 (TT)          FAX (301) 217-0968
e-mail: dsusa@dsusa.org           http://www.dsusa.org/ ~ dsusa/dsusa.html

In each of these videotapes, a person with the disability demonstrates a specially created exercise routine. 30 minutes each. Single title, $17.00; both titles on one videotape, $28.00; plus $4.50 shipping and handling.

Aging with Spinal Cord Injury
by Gale G. Whiteneck et al. (eds.)
Demos Vermande
386 Park Avenue South, Suite 201
New York, NY 10016
(800) 532-8663                    (212) 683-0072                 FAX (212) 683-0118

This book is an anthology of articles by a multidisciplinary group of experts in the field of spinal cord injury. Topics include research in the area of aging with a spinal cord injury, physiological and psychological aspects of the aging process, and societal perspectives. $99.95 plus $4.00 shipping and handling.

All Things are Possible
by Yvonne Duffy
A. J. Garvin and Associates
PO Box 7525
Ann Arbor, MI 48107

Written by a woman with a spinal cord injury, this book discusses issues specifically related to women, such as menstruation, childrearing, marriage, sex, and lesbianism. $8.95

The Body's Memory
by Jean Stewart
St. Martin's Press, New York, NY
Distributed by Publishers' Book and Audio
PO Box 070059
Staten Island, NY 10307
(800) 288-2131

A novel about a woman who must use a wheelchair as a result of surgery for removal of a tumor on her hip. Her story depicts relationships with colleagues, friends, and lovers, as well as her emotional upheaval and redefinition of her values. $10.95 plus $3.00 shipping and handling.

A Consumer's Guide to Home Adaptation
The Adaptive Environments Center
374 Congress Street, Suite 301
Boston, MA 02210
(617) 695-1225 (V/TT)

A workbook that enables people with mobility impairments to plan the modifications necessary to adapt their homes. Includes descriptions of widening doorways, lowering countertops, etc. $12.00

The Effect of Spinal Cord Injury on Female Sexuality
Medical Rehabilitation Research and Training Center in Prevention and Treatment of Secondary Complications of Spinal Cord Injury
Spain Rehabilitation Center
University of Alabama at Birmingham
1717 Sixth Avenue South, Room 506
Birmingham, AL 35233
(205) 934-3283          (205) 934-4642 (TT)          FAX (205) 975-4691
e-mail: Lindsey@sun.rehabm.uab.edu  http://www.sci.rehabm.uab.edu

This videotape, presented in lecture format, discusses how to attract and satisfy a partner, pleasuring and orgasm, intercourse, and pregnancy. 18 minutes. Purchase, $50.00; rental, $35.00.

Enabling Romance: A Guide to Love, Sex, and Relationships for the Disabled
by Ken Kroll and Erica Levy Klein
Woodbine House
6510 Bells Mill Road
Bethesda, MD 20817
(800) 843-7323          (301) 897-3570          FAX (301) 897-5838
e-mail: woodbine85@aol.com

Written by a man who has a disability and his wife who does not, this book provides examples of how people with a variety of disabilities, including spinal cord injuries, have established fulfilling relationships. Includes information about finding suitable partners and the use of personal attendants. $15.95 plus $4.00 shipping and handling.

Handicapped Moms - Mothers of Invention
Mary Free Bed Hospital and Rehabilitation Center
235 Wealthy Street, SE
Grand Rapids, MI 49503
(616) 242-0429                           (616) 454-3939

In this videotape, two women, one with a spinal cord injury, discuss the methods they have devised to raise their children and the barriers they have had to overcome. 9 minutes. Purchase, $165.00; rental for 10 working days, $35.00

The Impossible Takes a Little Longer
Instructional Support Services
Indiana University
601 East Kirkwood
Bloomington, IN 47405-1223
(800) 552-8620                    (812) 855-2103                    FAX (812) 855-8404

A videotape that profiles four women with disabilities, including one with paraplegia and one with quadriplegia, who have been successful in demanding professions and in family life. Deals with how they have handled insensitive reactions from the public. 46 minutes. Purchase, $170.00; rental, $35.00; plus $5.00 shipping and handling.

Intermittent Self-Catheterization
Media Services
Sacred Heart Medical Center
PO Box 2555
Spokane, WA 99220-2555
(509) 458-5236                    FAX (509) 626-4475

This videotape demonstrates the use of sterile techniques for intermittent catheterization and shows the necessary supplies and procedures. 8 minutes. Purchase, $135.00; rental for one week, $45.00 (may be applied toward purchase); plus $5.00 shipping and handling.

Journal of Rehabilitation Research and Development (JRRD)
Scientific and Technical Publications Section
Rehabilitation Research and Development Service
103 South Gay Street, 5th Floor
Baltimore, MD 21202
(410) 962-1800

A quarterly publication of scientific and engineering articles related to spinal cord injury, prosthetics and orthotics, sensory aids, and gerontology. Includes abstracts of literature, book reviews, and calendar of events. A special issue on choosing a wheelchair system appeared as Clinical Supplement # 2 to the March, 1990 edition. Free

Just What Can You Do?
Multi-Focus
1525 Franklin Street
San Francisco, CA 94109
(800) 821-0514                              (415) 673-5100

A discussion among four individuals with spinal cord injury, including one woman, this videotape includes information about sexuality, marriage, incontinence, attitudes, and personal experiences. 23 minutes. Videotape, $220.00; 16mm film, purchase, $450.00; rent, $60.00.

Keep Fit While You Sit
The Disability Bookshop
PO Box 129
Vancouver, WA 98666-0129
(800) 637-2256                              (206) 694-2462

This videotape demonstrates aerobic exercises for the arms, torso, neck, and shoulders for individuals who have no use of their lower body. 45 minutes. $29.95 plus $5.00 shipping and handling.

Key Changes
Fanlight Productions
47 Halifax Street
Boston, MA 02130
(800) 937-4113                (617) 542-0980               FAX (617) 542-8838
e-mail: fanlight@tiac.net     http://www.fanlight.com

This videotape portrays Lisa Thorson, a vocalist who experienced a spinal cord injury and continues performing in her chosen profession. 28 minutes. Purchase, $195.00; rental, $50.00; plus $9.00 shipping and handling.

Learning about Catheterization - Female
Medical Center of Vermont, Rehabilitation Center
111 Colchester Avenue
Burlington, VT 05401
(802) 656-5387                FAX (802) 656-2389

In this videotape, self-catheterization is demonstrated, and women with spinal cord injuries discuss their concerns about bladder problems. 19 minutes. Purchase, $65.00.

Living with Spinal Cord Injury
by Barry Corbett
Fanlight Productions
47 Halifax Street
Boston, MA 02130
(800) 937-4113                (617) 542-0980               FAX (617) 542-8838
e-mail: fanlight@tiac.net     http://www.fanlight.com

A series of three videotapes produced by an individual who has experienced spinal cord injury himself. "Changes" is about the consequences of spinal cord injury and the process of rehabilitation. "Outside" emphasizes the life-long aspect of rehabilitation for people with spinal cord injuries. "Survivors" interviews 23 men and women who have lived at least 24 years with spinal cord injuries. Purchase of single videotape, $125.00; rental for one day, $50.00; rental for one week, $100.00; $9.00 shipping and handling. Purchase of series, $250.00; call for shipping and handling.

Managing Incontinence
Cheryle B. Gartley, (ed.)
Simon Foundation for Continence
PO Box 815
Wilmette, IL 60091
(800) 237-4666                    (708) 864-3913                    FAX (708) 864-9758

This book provides medical advice, information on products, interviews with individuals who are incontinent, and advice on sexuality. $11.95

Mother-to-Be: A Guide to Pregnancy and Birth For Women with Disabilities
by Judith Rogers and Molleen Matsumura
Demos Vermande
386 Park Avenue South, Suite 201
New York, NY 10016
(800) 532-8663                    (212) 683-0072                    FAX (212) 683-0118

This book describes the pregnancy and childbirth experiences of 36 women with a wide variety of disabilities including spinal cord injury. Suggests practical solutions for the special concerns of women with disabilities during pregnancy and those of their partners, families, and health care providers. Includes a list of resources, glossary, and bibliography. $24.95 plus $4.00 shipping and handling.

National Database of Educational Resources on Spinal Cord Injury
The Institute for Rehabilitation and Research (TIRR)
Division of Education
1333 Moursund
Houston, TX 77030
(713) 797-5945                    (713) 797-5970 (TT)                    FAX (713) 797-5982
e-mail: lherson@bcm.tmc.edu

This database of publications, audiocassettes, and videotapes on spinal cord injury covers topics such as environmental modifications and accessibility, adaptive equipment and aids, vocational management, and recreation and leisure. Printouts for up to two subject areas are free. Complete database of both audio-visual materials and unpublished written materials, $50.00 plus $5.00 shipping and handling.

Paraplegia News
2111 East Highland Avenue, Suite 180
Phoenix, AZ 85016
(602) 224-0500

A monthly magazine sponsored by the Paralyzed Veterans of America. Features information for paralyzed veterans and civilians, articles about everyday living, new legislation, employment, and research. U.S., $21.00; foreign, $30.00.

Partners in Independence: The Personal Care Attendant's Role in Pressure Sore Prevention
The Institute for Rehabilitation and Research (TIRR)
Division of Education, B 107
1333 Moursund
Houston, TX 77030
(713) 797-5945                    (713) 797-5790 (TT)              FAX (713) 797-5982
e-mail: lherson@bcm.tmc.edu

A videotape that teaches how to detect skin problems and how to prevent them. 12 minutes. Available in English and Spanish. Consumers, $30.00; professionals, $85.00; plus $2.00 shipping and handling.

Physical Fitness: A Guide for Individuals with Spinal Cord Injury
by David F. Apple, Jr.
Scientific and Technical Publications Section
Rehabilitation Research and Development Service
103 South Gay Street, 5th Floor
Baltimore, MD 21202
(410) 962-1800

This anthology of articles written by a multidisciplinary group of professionals includes information about exercise tolerance and the development of specific fitness programs. Free

Positive Images
Women Make Movies
462 Broadway, Suite 500 E
New York, NY 10013
(212) 925-0606                    FAX (212) 925-2052              e-mail: orders@wmm.com

In this videotape, three women, including one with a spinal cord injury, discuss their lives at home, at work, and with family and friends. 58 minutes. Purchase, $295.00; rental for three days, $75.00; plus $15.00 shipping and handling.

Preventing Secondary Medical Complications: A Guide for Personal Assistants Working for People with Spinal Cord Injuries
Medical Rehabilitation Research and Training Center in Prevention and Treatment of Secondary Complications of Spinal Cord Injury
Spain Rehabilitation Center
University of Alabama at Birmingham
1717 Sixth Avenue South, Room 506
Birmingham, AL 35233
(205) 934-3283                    (205) 934-4642 (TT)              FAX (205) 975-4691
e-mail: Lindsey@sun.rehabm.uab.edu  http://www.sci.rehabm.uab.edu

This booklet provides training in the proper health care for people with spinal cord injury with an emphasis on daily routines. $3.50 plus $2.50 shipping and handling.

Reproductive Issues for Persons with Physical Disabilities
by Florence P. Haseltine, Sandra S. Cole, and David B. Gray (eds.)
Brookes Publishing Company
PO Box 10624
Baltimore, MD 21285-9945
(800) 638-3775                     e-mail: custserv@p.brookes.com

This book provides an overview of sexuality, disability, and reproductive issues across the lifespan for individuals with disabilities including spinal cord injuries. Includes academic articles as well as personal narratives written by individuals with disabilities. $34.00

Sexuality after Spinal Cord Injury: Answers to Your Questions
by Stanley H. Ducharme and Kathleen M. Gill
Brookes Publishing Company
PO Box 10624
Baltimore, MD 21285-9945
(800) 638-3775                     e-mail: custserv@p.brookes.com

Written by two clinical psychologists, this book addresses the questions faced by individuals after spinal cord injury, including social, psychological, and physical issues related to sexuality. $22.00

Sexuality Reborn
Education Department
Kessler Institute for Rehabilitation
1199 Pleasant Valley Way
West Orange, NJ 07052
(800) 435-8866

A videotape in which four couples, including one woman with spina bifida who uses a wheelchair for mobility, discuss the physical and emotional aspects of spinal cord injury upon their sex lives, including dating, bowel and bladder control, sexual response, and sexual activity. $39.95 plus $8.00 shipping and handling.

Spinal Cord Injury: A Manual for Healthy Living
The Institute for Rehabilitation Research (TIRR)
1333 Moursund
Houston, TX 77030
(713) 797-5946                     (713) 797-5790 (TT)                     FAX (713) 797-5982
e-mail: lherson@bcm.tmc.edu

This manual provides information on how to prevent complications associated with spinal cord injury. Includes information on skin care, sexuality, exercises, equipment, and more. Available in English and Spanish. $60.00 plus $2.00 shipping and handling.

Spinal Cord Injury Home Care Manual
Rehabilitation Educational Fund, Attn: Ellie Farzamian
Santa Clara Valley Medical Center
751 South Bascom Avenue
San Jose, CA 95128-2699
(408) 885-4010                         FAX (408) 885-4008

Provides people with spinal cord injuries, their families, and professionals with information about physical care, independent living, psychosocial issues, attendant care, and supplies.  $150.00

Spinal Cord Injury Resource Guide
National Rehabilitation Information Center (NARIC)
8455 Colesville Road, Suite 935
Silver Spring, MD 20910-3319
(800) 346-2742                    (301) 588-9284                    (301) 495-5626 (TT)
FAX (301) 587-1967               e-mail: naric@capaccess.org
http://www.naric.com/naric

This booklet lists sources of information about organizations, research, and publications related to spinal cord injury.  Includes information about recreational activities, special information for children, and information about sexuality.  Available online at NARIC's World Wide Web site and in standard print, large print, braille, and on computer disk.  Free

Spinal Cord Injury Self-Care Manual
Education Department
Shriners Hospital
1701 19th Avenue
San Francisco, CA 94122
(415) 665-1100

A manual that describes the medical aspects and complications of spinal cord injury, applicable services such as physical, occupational, and recreational therapy, sexuality, attendant care, and equipment.  Available in English and Spanish.  $50.00

Spinal Network
by Sam Maddox
Miramar Communications
PO Box 8987
Malibu, CA 90265
(800) 543-4116                    (310) 317-4522                    FAX (310) 317-9644

This book describes the medical aspects of spinal cord injury and the wide variety of its effects on functioning.  Presents biographical accounts of people who have lived with spinal cord injuries.  Discusses issues of everyday living, including recreation and sports, travel, and legal and financial concerns.  Softcover, $37.95; ring binder, $39.95; plus $6.00 shipping and handling.  "New Mobility" is a monthly magazine with updated information and articles on similar topics.  $37.95

Sports 'N Spokes
2111 East Highland Avenue, Suite 180
Phoenix, AZ 85016-9611
(602) 224-0500

A bimonthly magazine that features articles about sports activities for people who use wheelchairs.
U.S., $18.00; foreign, $21.00.

Substance Abuse in Rehabilitation Facilities - No Problem? Think Again...
The Institute for Rehabilitation and Research (TIRR)
Division of Education, B 107
1333 Moursund
Houston, TX 77030
(713) 797-5945                    (713) 797-5790 (TT)               FAX (713) 797-5982
e-mail: lherson@bcm.tmc.edu

In this videotape, a psychiatrist moderates a discussion by a panel of individuals with spinal cord
injuries who experienced substance abuse while in rehabilitation.  The role of the institution staff is
also discussed.  38 minutes.  $89.95 plus $2.00 shipping and handling.

Toward Independence: Considerations in Wheelchair Seating
Toward Independence: Female Quadriplegia Dressing
Mobility Research and Assessment Laboratory
University of Texas Southwest Medical Center
9705 Harry Hines avenue, Suite 105
Dallas, TX 75220-5441
(214) 351-2041

The first videotape discusses skin problems associated with wheelchair seating and suggests solutions.
In the second videotape, women with quadriplegia discuss how they learned dressing skills and used
adaptive techniques and clothing.  30 minutes each.  Either video, purchase, $250.00; rental $50.00.

# INDEX OF ORGANIZATIONS

This index contains only those organizations listed under sections titled "ORGANIZATIONS." These organizations may also be listed as vendors of publications, tapes, and other products.

# Publications from Resources for Rehabilitation

## A Woman's Guide to Coping with Disability

This <u>unique</u> book addresses the special needs of women with disabilities and chronic conditions, such as social relationships, sexual functioning, pregnancy, childrearing, caregiving, and employment. Special attention is paid to ways in which women can advocate for their rights with the health care and rehabilitation systems. Written for women in all age categories, the book has chapters on the disabilities that are most prevalent in women or likely to affect the roles and physical functions unique to women. Included are arthritis, diabetes, epilepsy, lupus, multiple sclerosis, osteoporosis, and spinal cord injury. Each chapter also includes information about the condition, professional service providers, and psychological aspects plus descriptions of organizations, publications and tapes, and special assistive devices. This new edition includes e-mail addresses and Internet resources.

Second edition, 1997                                ISBN 0-929718-19-4     $42.95

*Chosen by **Library Journal** as a book of outstanding quality and significance. "...this excellent, empowering resource belongs in all collections."*

*"...crucial information women need to be informed, empowered, and in control of their lives. Excellent self-help information... **Highly recommended** for public and academic libraries." **Choice***

*"...a marvelous publication...will help women feel more in control of their lives." **A nurse who became disabled***

## A Man's Guide to Coping with Disability

Written to fill the void in the literature regarding the special needs of men with disabilities, this book includes information about men's responses to disability, with a special emphasis on the values men place on independence, occupational achievement, and physical activity. Information on finding local services, self-help groups, laws that affect men with disabilities, sports and recreation, and employment is applicable to men with any type of disability or chronic condition. The disabilities that are most prevalent in men or that affect men's special roles in society are included. Chapters on coronary heart disease, diabetes, HIV/AIDS, multiple sclerosis, prostate conditions, spinal cord injury, and stroke include information about the disease or condition, psychological aspects, sexual functioning, where to find services, environmental adaptations, and annotated entries of organizations, publications and tapes, and resources for assistive devices. Includes e-mail addresses and Internet resources.

1997                                                ISBN 0-929718-18-6     $42.95

*"a unique reference source." **Library Journal***
*"a unique purchase for public libraries" **Booklist/Reference Books Bulletin***

## Resources for Elders with Disabilities

This book meets the needs of elders, family members, and other caregivers. Published in LARGE PRINT (**18 point bold type**), the book provides information about rehabilitation, laws that affect elders with disabilities, and self-help groups. Each chapter that deals with a specific disability or condition has information on the causes and treatments for the condition; psychological aspects; professional service providers; where to find services; environmental adaptations; and suggestions for making everyday living safer and easier. Chapters on hearing loss, vision loss, Parkinson's disease, stroke, arthritis, osteoporosis, and diabetes also provide information on organizations, publications and tapes, and assistive devices. Throughout the book are practical suggestions to prevent accidents and to facilitate interactions with family members, friends, and service providers. Plus information about aids for everyday living, older workers, falls, travel, and housing.

Third edition, 1996                                ISBN 0-929718-16-X     $48.95

*"...especially useful for older readers. **Highly recommended.**" **Library Journal***
*"...a valuable, well organized, easy-to-read reference source." **American Reference Books Annual***
*"...a handy ready-reference..."                **Reference Books Bulletin/Booklist***

## Meeting the Needs of Employees with Disabilities

This resource guide provides the information people with disabilities need to retain or obtain employment. Includes information on government programs and laws such as the Americans with Disabilities Act, training programs, supported employment, transition from school to work, assistive technology, and environmental adaptations. Chapters on hearing and speech impairments, mobility impairments, and visual impairment and blindness describe organizations, adaptive equipment, and services plus suggestions for a safe and friendly workplace. Case vignettes describing accommodations for employees with disabilities are a new special feature.

Second edition, 1993                                    ISBN 0-929718-13-5     $42.95

*"...a valuable resource...for professionals and human resources personnel..."*
                              *Journal of Applied Rehabilitation Counseling*
*"...solid and up-to-date."*      *Journal of Career Planning and Employment*
*"...an **excellent** directory for those challenged with incorporating persons with disabilities in the workplace..."*
                              *AAOHN Journal*
*"...recommended for public libraries and for academic libraries..."*
                              *Choice*
*"...a **timely** resource...Libraries with a focus on disabilities or employment issues will want the book... RQ*
*"...this book is **unique**...an **important** acquisition..."*
                              *American Reference Books Annual*

## Living with Low Vision: A Resource Guide for People with Sight Loss

This LARGE PRINT (**18 point bold type**) comprehensive guide helps people with sight loss locate the services, products, and publications that they need to keep reading, working, and enjoying life. Chapters for children and elders plus information on self-help groups, how to keep reading and working with vision loss, and making everyday living easier. Information on laws that affect people with vision loss, including the ADA, and high tech equipment that promotes independence and employment. Includes e-mail addresses and Internet resources.

Fourth edition, 1996                                    ISBN 0-929718-14-3     $43.95

*"No other complete resource guide exists..an **invaluable** tool for locating services.. for public and academic libraries."*
                              *Library Journal*
*"...a **good** reference for libraries serving visually handicapped individuals."*
                              *American Reference Books Annual*
*"...a **very** useful resource for patients experiencing vision loss."*   *Archives of Ophthalmology*
*"...a **superb** resource...should be made available in waiting rooms or patient education areas..."*
                              *American Journal of Ophthalmology*
*"This volume is a **treasure chest** of concise, useful information."*       *OT Week*

## Resources for People with Disabilities and Chronic Conditions

This comprehensive resource guide has chapters on spinal cord injury, low back pain, diabetes, multiple sclerosis, hearing and speech impairments, vision impairment and blindness, and epilepsy. Each chapter includes information about the disease or condition; psychological aspects of the condition; professional service providers; environmental adaptations; assistive devices; and descriptions of organizations, publications, and products. Chapters on rehabilitation services, independent living, self-help, laws that affect people with disabilities (including the ADA), and making everyday living easier. Special information for children is also included. Includes e-mail addresses and Internet resources. Third edition, 1996                    ISBN 0-929718-17-8     $49.95

*"...**wide** coverage and **excellent** organization of this **encyclopedic** guide...recommended..."* Choice
*"**Sensitive** to the tremendous variety of needs and circumstances of living with a disability."*       *American Libraries*
*"...an **excellent** resource for consumers and professionals..."* *Journal of the American Paraplegia Society*
*"...improves the chances of library patrons finding needed services..."* *American Reference Books Annual*
*"...an **excellent** reference that should be in every family physician's office as well as in libraries..."*
                              *Journal of the American Board of Family Physicians*

## LARGE PRINT PUBLICATIONS

**_Designed for distribution by professionals to people with disabilities and chronic conditions_**

These publications serve as self-help guides for people with disabilities and chronic conditions. They include information on the condition, rehabilitation services, products, and resources that contribute to independence. Titles include **Living with Hearing Loss, Living with Arthritis, After a Stroke, Living with Diabetes, Aging and Vision Loss, Living with Low Vision,** and **How to Keep Reading with Vision Loss.**

8 1/2" by 11"   Printed in **18 point bold type** on ivory paper with black ink for maximum contrast.

_"These are **exciting products**. We look forward to doing business with you again."   A rehabilitation professional_

### Rehabilitation Resource Manual: VISION

A desk reference that enables service providers, librarians, and others to make effective referrals. Includes guidelines on starting self-help groups; information on professional research and service organizations; plus chapters on assistive technology; for special populations; and by eye condition/disease.   Case vignettes demonstrating multidisciplinary cooperation in providing services to people with vision loss are a new special feature of the Manual. Updated address list included.

Fourth edition, 1993                                       ISBN 0-929718-10-0     $39.95

_"...the best ready-access source available in this field."   OT Week_
_"The book will be of great use in the ophthalmologist's office."       American Journal of Ophthalmology_
_"...should be a part of every eye care professional/service provider library."   Journal of Rehabilitation_

### Providing Services for People with Vision Loss:  A Multidisciplinary Perspective
#### Susan L. Greenblatt, Editor

Written by ophthalmologists, rehabilitation professionals, a physician who has experienced vision loss, and a sociologist, this book discusses how various professionals can work together to provide coordinated care for people with vision loss. Chapters include Vision Loss: A Patient's Perspective; Vision Loss: An Ophthalmologist's Perspective;  Operating a Low Vision Aids Service;  The Need for Coordinated Care;  Making Referrals for Rehabilitation Services;  Mental Health Services: The Missing Link; Self-Help Groups  for People with Sight Loss; and Aids and Techniques that Help People with Vision Loss plus a Glossary.  Also available on cassette.

1989                                                  ISBN 0-929718-02-X    $19.95

_"...an **excellent** overview of the perspectives and clinical services that facilitate rehabilitation."_
                                    _Archives of Ophthalmology_
_"...an **excellent** guide for professionals."   Journal of Rehabilitation_

### Meeting the Needs of People with Vision Loss:  A Multidisciplinary Perspective
#### Susan L. Greenblatt, Editor

Written by rehabilitation professionals, physicians, and a sociologist, this book discusses how to provide appropriate information and how to serve special populations. Chapters include What People with Vision Loss Need to Know; Information and Referral Services for People with Vision Loss; The Role of the Family in the Adjustment to Blindness or Visual Impairment; Diabetes and Vision Loss - Special Considerations; Special Needs of Children and Adolescents; Older Adults with Vision and Hearing Losses; Providing Services to Visually Impaired Elders in Long Term Care Facilities; plus a series of Multidisciplinary Case Studies. Also available on cassette.

1991                                                  ISBN 0-929718-07-0    $24.95

_"...of use to anyone concerned with improving service delivery to the growing population of people who are visually impaired."                    American Journal of Occupational Therapy_

# RESOURCES for REHABILITATION

33 Bedford Street, Suite 19A • Lexington, MA 02173 • 617-862-6455   FAX 617-861-7517

*Our Federal Employer Identification Number is 04-2975-007*

NAME _____

ORGANIZATION _____

ADDRESS _____

PHONE _____

[ ] Check or signed institutional purchase order enclosed for full amount of order.  Purchase orders accepted from government agencies, hospitals, and universities <u>only</u>.

[ ] Mastercard/VISA Card number: _____

Signature: _____Expiration date: _____

### ALL ORDERS OF $100.00 OR LESS <u>MUST</u> BE PREPAID.

| TITLE | QUANTITY | PRICE | TOTAL |
|---|---|---|---|
| A Woman's Guide to Coping with Disability | ____ X | $42.95 | ____ |
| A Man's Guide to Coping with Disability | ____ X | 42.95 | ____ |
| Resources for People with Disabilities and Chronic Conditions | ____ X | 49.95 | ____ |
| Resources for Elders with Disabilities | ____ X | 48.95 | ____ |
| Living with Low Vision:  A Resource Guide | ____ X | 43.95 | ____ |
| Rehabilitation Resource Manual:  VISION | ____ X | 39.95 | ____ |
| Meeting the Needs of Employees with Disabilities | ____ X | 42.95 | ____ |
| Providing Services for People with Vision Loss | ____ X | 19.95 | ____ |
|    [ ] Check here for audiocassette edition | | | |
| Meeting the Needs of People with Vision Loss | ____ X | 24.95 | ____ |
|    [ ] Check here for audiocassette edition | | | |

### <u>MINIMUM PURCHASE OF 25 COPIES PER TITLE FOR THE FOLLOWING PUBLICATIONS</u>

Call for discount on purchases of 100 or more copies of any single title.

| | QUANTITY | PRICE | TOTAL |
|---|---|---|---|
| After a stroke | ____ X | 1.75 | ____ |
| Living with diabetes | ____ X | 1.50 | ____ |
| Living with low vision | ____ X | 2.00 | ____ |
| How to keep reading with vision loss | ____ X | 1.75 | ____ |
| Aging and vision loss | ____ X | 1.25 | ____ |
| Living with age-related macular degeneration | ____ X | 1.25 | ____ |
| Aids for everyday living with vision loss | ____ X | 1.25 | ____ |
| Living with diabetic retinopathy | ____ X | 1.75 | ____ |
| High tech aids for people with vision loss | ____ X | 1.75 | ____ |
| Living with arthritis | ____ X | 1.50 | ____ |
| Living with hearing loss | ____ X | 1.50 | ____ |
| | SUB-TOTAL | | ____ |

SHIPPING & HANDLING: $50.00 or less, add $5.00; $50.01 to 100.00, add $8.00; add $4.00 for each additional $100.00 or fraction of $100.00.  Alaska, Hawaii, U.S. territories, and Canada, add $3.00 to shipping and handling charges

Foreign orders must be prepaid in U.S. currency.  Please write for shipping charges.

<u>*Prices are subject to change.*</u>

SHIPPING/HANDLING _____

TOTAL                    $_____